Rolling On

The Story of the Amazing Gary McPherson

For Nick,

A small token of appreciation.

March 3/07   Gerald

Rolling On

The Story of the Amazing
Gary McPherson

GERALD W. HANKINS

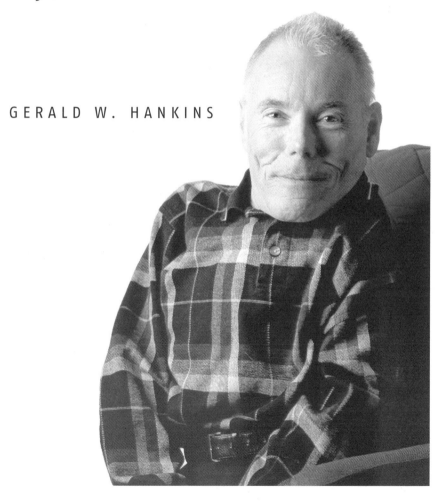

The University of Alberta Press

Published by

The University of Alberta Press
Ring House 2
Edmonton, Alberta, Canada T6G 2E1

Copyright © Gerald W. Hankins 2003

NATIONAL LIBRARY OF CANADA
CATALOGUING IN PUBLICATION

Hankins, Gerald W.
    Rolling on : the story of the amazing
    Gary McPherson /
    author, Gerald W. Hankins.

    Includes bibliographical references.
    ISBN 0-88864-405-1

    1. McPherson, Gary, 1946- —Health.
2. Quadriplegics—Alberta—Biography.
3. Poliomyelitis—Patients—Alberta—
Biography. I. Title.

RC406.Q33H35 2003   362.4'3'092
C2003-905730-5

Printed and bound in Canada by Houghton
Boston Printers, Saskatoon, Saskatchewan
First edition, first printing, 2003
All rights reserved.

The University of Alberta Press is committed
to protecting our natural environment. As
part of our efforts, this book is printed on
New Leaf Paper: it contains 100% post-
consumer recycled fibres and is acid- and
chlorine-free.

The University of Alberta Press gratefully
acknowledges the support received for its
publishing program from The Canada
Council for the Arts. The University of
Alberta Press also gratefully acknowledges
the financial support of the Government of
Canada through the Book Publishing
Industry Development Program (BPIDP) and
from the Alberta Foundation for the Arts for
its publishing activities.

Canadä

To Val McPherson and two great kids, Keiko and Jamie McPherson.

You know, sometimes it is the artist's task to find out how much music you can still make with what you have left.

—ITZHAK PERLMAN

Virtuoso and polio survivor, at the conclusion of a violin concerto on November 18, 1995, at the Lincoln Center, New York. After a string snapped early in the performance, he paused briefly, then carried on playing to the end.

Contents

Foreword

From Abandonment to Inclusion

MOST OF THE IMPORTANT CHANGES in the recognition of the rights of persons with disability have occurred during Dr. Gary McPherson's lifetime. Today, in contrast to relatively recent history, persons with disability can often look forward to "normal" and, in some cases, longer lives, with full participation in an inclusive society. It was not always this way. Historically, attitudes towards persons with disability were fundamentally negative, characterized by abandonment, persecution, institutionalization, segregation and marginalization. Only during the last half-century have persons with disability begun to enjoy the same rights as so-called able-bodied persons.

World wars, other conflicts and disease have left millions of persons with physical, sensory, emotional and intellectual disabilities. The polio epidemic of the 1950s alone left thousands of persons with severe disability.

The Universal Declaration of Human Rights recognizes the rights of all persons in society, and disability-specific initiatives such as the International Year of the Disabled, the Decade of the Disabled and the International Day of the Disabled have raised world consciousness regarding the issues and rights of persons with disability. The UN Standard Rules of Equalization of Opportunity for Persons with Disabilities challenged governments to provide equal opportunities. Various governments now legislate the rights of adults and children with disability.

In Canada, the Charter of Human Rights and Freedoms (1982) specifically highlights the rights of persons with disability. The formation of the International Paralympic Committee in 1989 brought elite disability sport and athletes with disability into the mainstream. Elite disability sport fundamentally challenged the assumptions of disease, DISability, dependence and charitable condescension. Finally, the World Health Organization's shift from the International Classification of Impairments, Disabilities and Handicaps (1980) to the International Classification of Functioning, Disability and Health (2001) altered the disability paradigm from person-centred to context- or environment-centred.

We have progressed from segregation and institutionalization to the concept of inclusion—which recognizes the rights of persons with disability to be fully participatory members of society in all aspects of daily living, and to access the necessary support systems and services.

Gary McPherson has lived through most of these changes and now is an agent of change himself. Institutionalized as a result of the polio epidemic in the 1950s, he was deprived of the degree of personal freedom and physical ability ordinarily enjoyed by youth and adolescents. Advances in human rights initiatives, improvements to home care, and transformed attitudes towards disability have provided an environment today which frees him to access opportunity and demonstrate his true abilities.

Through changes in care for and the rights of persons with disabilities, Gary found the space and freedom to influence the values and philosophies that for so long had restricted his opportunities and freedoms. He has been, and remains, a significant influence in changing societal attitudes and disability rights, as his former roles as chair of the Premier's Council on the Status of Persons with Disabilities and president of the Canadian Wheelchair Sports Association, and now as an educator at the University of Alberta, along with countless other initiatives bear witness.

Yet Gary is an exceptional character, and it would be naïve to suggest that we have "made it"—that persons with disability are, without exception, fully included participating members of society. There remains much to be done. Advocacy on behalf of persons with disability will continue to be important, as will a broader understanding of what *inclusion* really means and implies.

In conclusion, consider Al Condeluci's words:

Inclusion means being at the table; being part of the discourse; being respected for who you are....Inclusion acknowledges that people may be different and pushes us to respect that diversity. It is a term that implies welcoming to all...we need to understand that inclusion is much more than just being in a group. It is comprised of all the deep and important relationship elements that makes us feel welcomed and at home with that group. —*Beyond Difference*, 1996

The energy, insight, wisdom and humanity that distinguish Dr. Gary McPherson are the threads through which societal attitudes and values will continue to weave a tapestry of change.

ROBERT D. STEADWARD

O.C., Ph.D., LL.D. (Hon.)
Professor Emeritus, University of Alberta
Founder and CEO, Steadward Centre for Personal and Physical Achievement
Founding, Past and Honorary President, International Paralympic Committee

GARRY D. WHEELER

Ph.D., C. Psych.
Adjunct Professor, University of Alberta
Manager of Research and Counselling, Steadward Centre

Preface
University Honors

IT SEEMED LIKE ALL OF EDMONTON was streaming towards the Jubilee Auditorium on Thursday, November 16, 1995, for the University of Alberta's fall convocation. My wife Alison and I were among the crowd milling around the foyer and then scrambling for seats inside. We had driven up to Edmonton to attend our daughter Jennifer's graduation in nursing. When the band played the processional signalling the arrival of the chancellor and members of the platform party, we and everyone else in the audience rose from our seats as they slowly made their way towards the front and onto the stage.

From where I sat high up on the balcony, one member of the platform party looked strangely out of place.

There he was, sitting comfortably in his wheelchair among the academic elite of the University of Alberta. His repetitive facial grimaces were odd—certainly signs of something abnormal within, I thought. He gave the appearance of having a mouthful of sticky toffee. I had to wait almost two hours to satisfy my curiosity.

In the meantime, some 760 capped-and-gowned graduating students paraded across the platform. Chancellor Lou Hyndman, garbed in the magnificent blue gown of his office, shook the hand of each one, and

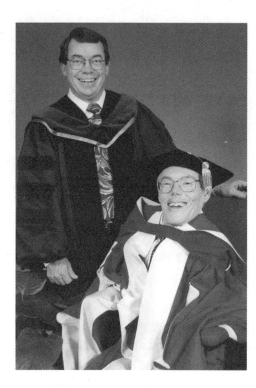

Presented by Dr. Robert Steadward, Dr. Gary McPherson received an Honorary Doctor of Laws Degree in recognition of his significant contribution to the community by the University of Alberta Senate.

The University of Alberta

President Rod Fraser, wearing the traditional green and gold of the university, greeted and congratulated the graduands.

Then Dr. Robert Steadward, professor of physical education and recreation, and chair of the International Paralympic Committee, introduced the man with the wheelchair. Not only was he to be presented with an Honorary Doctor of Laws, he also had been given the awesome task of delivering the convocation address.

When Dr. Steadward introduced Gary McPherson as "adjunct professor, community volunteer, provincial administrator and proactive crusader for the rights and betterment of people with a disability throughout the world," I began to realize how wrong my first impressions were. He went on to describe Gary as someone who "exemplifies the very finest qualities in a human being: concern, commitment, enthusiasm, initiative, diplomacy, compassion, pride and integrity." As the hood for the honorary degree fell over his shoulders, Gary was greeted with thunderous applause, the audience standing to acknowledge this man who would never be able to stand again.

Gary gave an inspiring address, filled with wit and wisdom. Early on, he answered the question: why the odd grimaces? In years long past, he explained, a disease had paralyzed his limbs and breathing muscles. To compensate, he had learned how to do glossopharyngeal breathing, also known as "frog-breathing." By opening his mouth and then gulping in air, he could force air down his windpipe.

Gary went on to say that receiving an honorary degree from a prestigious university did not necessarily confer a corresponding respect from his family and friends. In order to be properly fitted with a cap and gown, he had asked his wife to measure the circumference of his head. When he asked her what size it was, she quietly muttered, "It's getting bigger." And meanwhile, in the backyard, a neighbour was conversing with Gary's son, Jamie, saying that his dad was a pretty important man. After a long silence, Jamie replied, "I'm four and a half!"

Now associated with the University of Alberta for a number of years, Gary McPherson was then, in 1995, chairperson of the Premier's Council on the Status of Persons with Disabilities, spanning six hundred organizations. His contributions on behalf of the disabled have been outstanding.

During his thirty-four years of being confined in institutions and imprisoned in a severely disabled body, Gary found that if he had the right attitude and motivation, he could do all sorts of things. Most of his schooling came from correspondence courses; his real education, from everyday life. Dependency on others for most of his daily needs proved to be a great teacher. He learned to respect and be prepared to learn from everyone he met. He tried to be as active as he could, within the limitations of his disability, and to learn as much as he could in order to be a fully participating member of society.

Describing his wheelchair as "a tremendously liberating tool," he seemed to personify freedom from the restraints that hold so many people back.

In his convocation speech, he counselled the graduands to commit themselves to a process of continuous learning, as "the microchip is causing information and knowledge to double every eighteen months." As one who had looked into the face of adversity for most of his life, he felt comfortable suggesting that his audience turn adversity into something positive by "taking the lessons it teaches us and applying them in our lives for the benefit of ourselves and others." Further, he advised, adversity can put us in touch with the deepest part of our being—our soul and our spirit.

When Gary concluded his address, the crowd in the jam-packed Jubilee Auditorium had learned a lot more besides what frog-breathing was. In appreciation, they rose to their feet a second time in tribute to a man who had overcome great adversity and remained thankful for life.

On this day in 1995, I first met Gary McPherson. What follows is the story of his remarkable life and career.

GERALD W. HANKINS

August 2003

Acknowledgements

THE WRITING OF MOST BOOKS is a team effort and *Rolling On* is no exception. The author feels indebted to a great number of people.

A more cooperative subject than Gary McPherson would be hard to find. His and Val's welcoming home in the Riverbend district of Edmonton became familiar territory to me.

Special people who helped unearth ancient and recent pictures and clippings were Dorothy McPherson, Janet Tkachyk (nee Ross), and Connie Packer. Photographs not credited came from Gary's family. My apologies for any omissions.

I am happy to give thanks to Glenn Rollans for suggesting the title *Rolling On*. Paul Baker and Helen Huston supplied the details about Itzhak Perlman's feat with only three strings on his violin.

I appreciate the careful and detailed introduction written by Dr. Bob Steadward and Dr. Garry Wheeler. I want to thank Ralph Klein, Rick Hansen and Ray Cohen for their comments for the book cover.

I have been blessed with fine editors. Marcia Laycock, an experienced writer from Ponoka, was the first to see areas needing improvement and re-arranging. Thank you, Marcia. I have never met Jill Fallis from Victoria but am certainly grateful for her painstaking checking for details and accuracy. I appreciate the work of the staff of the University of Alberta Press who applied the important finishing touches that precede publication.

The author is grateful for the assistance of the following people with whom he conducted over ninety personal interviews, in addition to a handful of telephone interviews and correspondence by letter or email, during the research period from 1996 to 2001: Ted Aaron, Jim Allen, Ray Allison, Joanne Bastarache (nee McPherson), Eric Boyd, Carlene Brenneis, Don Buchanan, Wendy Buckley, Russell Carr, Bob Chelmick, Marion Chomik, Ernie Daigle, George de Rappard, Randy Dickinson, Dwayne Doberthein, Jack Donohue (deceased), Peter Eriksson, Dan Fortin, Ron Fortin, Brent Foster, Betty Fraser, Bob Fraser, Charlie Gardner, Betty George, Don Getty, Lorraine Habekost, Frank Haley, Rick Hansen, Braden Hirsch, Doug Johnson, Kay Klepachek, William Lakey, Greg Latham, Walter Lawrence, Reg McClellan, Dorothy McPherson, Roderick McPherson, Valerie McPherson (nee Kamitomo), Keiko McPherson, Jamie McPherson, Dean Mellway, Al Menard, Vance Milligan, Ron Minor, Eric Newell, Louise Nkunzi, Chukwuemeka Obiajunwa, Gary Ogletree, Karen O'Neill, Fran Osokin, Connie Packer, Adrienne Riley, Brian Riley, Lea Sanderson, Carl Shields, Marshal Smith (deceased), Brian Sproule, Bob Steadward, Darlene Steljes, Cam Tait, Janet Tkachyk (nee Ross), Jim Vargo (deceased), Olga Warren, Gerry Way, Percy Wickman, Ron Willson, Kim Worth (nee McPherson) and Randy Wyness.

I would like to thank the Alberta Medical Foundation and John Kok of Navigator Financial for each providing a grant towards the costs of publication.

As always, my wife Alison has been most supportive and encouraging while secretly hoping (I think) that these "projects" will one day come to an end.

For the practical help and support of these and unnamed others, I am most grateful.

1 | A Day in the Life of Gary McPherson

"EVERY DAY IS A GOOD DAY," Gary McPherson once said, "and some days are better than others."

How is it possible for anyone to call every day a good one? How can it be possible for any day to be good when you're a quadriplegic? Where is the so-called quality of life that the proponents of euthanasia are always trumpeting? Able-bodied people are often baffled to hear people like Gary make such a claim. Having reached the age of fifty-five after surviving for forty-six years since being struck with poliomyelitis, what in his present day-to-day life enables him to make such an incredible statement?

To find out, one evening while we were discussing various matters I asked him to describe an "ordinary" day. "Gary, let's begin with night-time. During your waking hours, you've said that frog-breathing allows adequate respiration in place of your paralyzed diaphragm and chest muscles. How on earth do you manage to sleep when you can't breathe without doing that?"

"I use a ventilator, which does the breathing for me all night long. It has controls for the volume of air I get and the rate of respiration. The moisture from my expired air is collected and used again so that my breathing tubes don't dry out. A flexible tube runs from the ventilator to

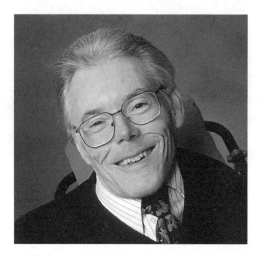

a mouthpiece that was custom-made for me by a dentist, and I'm thankful for it. With it in place and a good flow of air, I fall asleep feeling quite secure. It's quite a contrast from those terrible times when I was young and struggling for breath. I usually set the ventilator to cycle twelve times a minute at eight litres of air. Now I usually sleep about six hours without interruption, then doze off and on for another two hours."

"How does your day begin?"

"At 6:20 the clock-radio turns on. My wife, Val, gets up, separates me from the ventilator, then gives me a big glass of water to drink and a urine bottle before she goes out jogging, as she does three times a week. Around 6:45 Joanne White, my attendant, comes and brushes my teeth and dresses me in bed.

"Before lifting me out of bed, Joanne straps on my fibreglass brace that gives the support in place of my weakened back muscles. Someone has described my twisted back as looking like cooked spaghetti. Without the brace I couldn't sit up at all. It has to fit just right: tight enough to support my back without constricting breathing. Then I do my exercises."

"Exercises?"

"I sit in the wheelchair, and Joanne straps my feet to the pedals of the stationary bike. I have just enough strength in my left leg to keep both feet rotating. I have to keep the tension pretty low, but I do get some exercise. While on the bike, Val or my attendant mixes for me a glass of fruit juice with a scoop of protein powder and some other goodies and half a bagel, which I usually share with Chester, our little dog. It's a sort of workout that lasts about twenty minutes, and during that time I listen to audiotapes of an educational kind and sometimes to the CBC.

"Joanne puts me on the toilet by what I call a standing transfer and then gives me a shave. Then she lays me on a special shower platform— something I designed myself. It's like a wooden frame of cedar that sits firmly on the top of the bathtub and is hinged at the bottom end, allowing it to be raised. Narrow spaces between the slats allow water to drain into the tub. Joanne lays me down on the platform with my head near the tap. She washes my hair and then soaps and hoses my body with a hand-held shower, like a car wash. She then puts a towel under me and dries me off.

"She straps on my leg bag (some call it my pee-bag), which is hooked up to a condom catheter during the day. I can't quite handle a urinal, except at night. Then she dresses me, usually putting on a shirt, tie and jacket if I'm going out. Takes less than half an hour.

"In the meantime, whether I'm showering or exercising, Val is looking after the kids and getting them ready for school. The exercise routine is usually done by 8:20 when the time comes for Joanne and me to take Keiko and Jamie to school in our van, [which is] equipped with a hydrauli- cally operated wheelchair lift. If Val is not working, she drives them, since the school is some distance away. Then we'll head off to the univer- sity, or perhaps to a meeting somewhere. Sometimes I have an eight o'clock meeting and have to leave earlier. But if I don't have outside commitments, I'll stay at home and work on the computer. What I like best is a flexible program, and I don't mind working late or long as long as I can manage the time well."

"What are you doing at the university?"

"It varies. My time is not quite so tightly scheduled as it was for my old job at the Premier's Council [on the Status of Persons with Disabilities].

If our group is meeting, it'll be in the Faculty of Business or at the faculty club. A lot of the administrative work I can do from home on my computer. I've been trying to finish work at the university by 3:00 so that I can pick up the kids from school.

"I have a mobile office phone on my wheelchair, so I can field calls and make calls on the run. I have a tiny earplug and a mini-microphone three inches below my chin. The phone is on the armrest, and I can dial numbers with my left index finger. If I'm talking on the phone and another call comes in, it will automatically be recorded. At home I have another phone that I can activate with my knee, same effect as lifting the receiver. By my desk is a hand-held set with a speaker on it; when it rings I can answer by pushing a small button by my left hand."

"I understand that the computer has really changed your life."

"True, it has opened up my world since I got it in 1996. I feel fortunate that I can click the mouse with my left index finger. But since I can't operate the keyboard, I had to get the software for voice activation."

"Was it hard to get the computer to receive your voice messages properly?"

"It took months to do so, and it's still going on. Part of the problem is due to my breathing—sometimes I have more amplification than others. Then when the dog barks or the kids holler or Val drops a saucepan, the microphone on the computer picks up all those sounds. Sometimes the computer misinterprets a word. For example, I sent an e-mail to a friend expressing gratitude for her thoughtfulness in sending me a picture. The friend replied to my e-mail, expressing surprise that I considered her thoughtless. It took some apologizing. But once the computer gets the correct spelling, the word won't be misspelled again."

"You can't make notes on a piece of paper. How did you assemble all the thoughts and ideas for your book?"

"I read here and there, and if there's stuff I want to use or remember, I put it on the computer. Same for quotations I come across or interesting things on an audiotape. But if I'm out somewhere and get a sudden brainwave, I'll ask someone to write it down for me."

"You've got friends all across the country. You must have a constant stream of e-mail correspondence."

"Yes, I do. E-mail has allowed me to keep in touch with a lot of people, avoiding the need to buy and lick stamps or to get people to write letters for me. And I'm making fewer and fewer mistakes."

"You've got quite a reputation as a communicator. But how do you keep in touch with the outside world, current events and the likes?"

"I rely on the radio and the internet. Also the newspaper. I used to get people to pin a page of the paper on a line; I would read one side and then wheel around and read the other. Nowadays, if someone lays the paper on a corner of the table for me, I can lean forward in the wheelchair and with my left thumb and first finger slowly turn a page over. I need Val's help to get letters or papers or office material."

"You've said how important your family is to you. With all your many and varied activities, are you able to set aside the time for them that you'd like?"

"I try to give my family high priority, but I don't do as well as I should. The kids love to play knowledge games and some card games. We make a point of going to all the soccer games whenever [my daughter] Keiko's team is playing. And Val and I go out socially quite a lot."

"Getting back to your daily routine, what happens when Joanne goes home in the afternoon?"

"Val makes supper for us all, and she or one of the kids feeds me. At bedtime she brushes my teeth, washes my face, then undresses me and takes off my leg bag and condom catheter. Then she puts me to bed, kisses me goodnight and puts the mouthpiece in my mouth. This is her daily contribution, over and above the daily household duties. Val is very efficient. She is the pillar of my life."

During the course of an average day, Gary rarely thinks about having a disability—unless Val is at work, and his attendant is sick and unable to come that day. Then he is forcefully reminded what it means to be without the use of his arms or legs.

He believes in the importance of planning, but refuses to let tomorrow and its uncertainties and anxieties interfere with his work and enjoyment of today. He focuses on today, giving of his best towards current projects and always asking what he can do for his family. His everyday philosophy is echoed in the following three lines from the Sanskrit poem "Salutation to the Dawn":

Today well lived
Makes every Yesterday a dream of Happiness,
And every Tomorrow a vision of Hope.

2 | Schoolboy in the Yukon

"I REMEMBER HIM AS A YOUNG LAD with a great zest for living. A real self-starter. He was always the one to say, 'Let's go and play ball'."

So spoke Kay Klepachek, teacher of a one-room school in Swift River, Yukon Territory, about 180 kilometres (110 miles) from Watson Lake. Nine-year-old Gary McPherson was her pupil for less than a year in 1954–55, but he must have made a deep impression—forty-four years later the memories of him resurfaced with ease. Gary was a good student; in fact, Kay encouraged him to combine grades two and three in one year. He sailed through.

Kay also remembers Gary as "a determined boy with lots of confidence" who often organized games for the kids, even the older ones. He loved any kind of sports. "He may have been responsible, but he wasn't an angel," Gary's mother, Dorothy, confided. "He was mischievous and got into all kinds of scraps."

Kay Klepachek met the McPherson family when Gary's mother invited her to Sunday dinner the weekend before school started. After her marriage to Walter, they became regular visitors to the McPherson home. She was sorry when the family was transferred to Watson Lake some time in the spring.

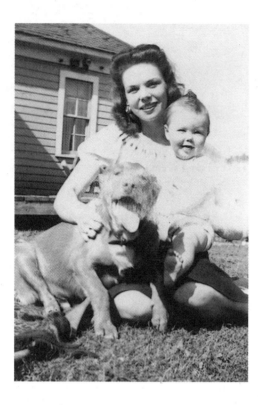

Dorothy Wilcox with her one year old son Gary and family pet "Timothy" in July, 1947.

Gary William Wilcox McPherson was born in Edson, Alberta, on June 28, 1946, the firstborn of David Lloyd Wilcox and Dorothy Florence Black. Dorothy, an Englishwoman, had met David, a sergeant in the Royal Canadian Engineers, at the Maple Leaf Club in London, England, near the end of the Second World War. They subsequently married, and six weeks later David was repatriated to Canada. Dorothy, aged twenty, followed him and landed in Edmonton in March 1946 before going to Edson, home of David's family. Two years later they moved to Edmonton, where another child, Joanne, was born.

Life was happy and uncomplicated for the Wilcox family until tragedy struck. In 1950, David died at the age of thirty-two from a massive heart attack. Dorothy was devastated. Now a young widow with two children under four, she was tempted to return to England, where she could count on support from family and friends. But, she said, "I loved Canada." She decided to stay, knowing full well it would be a risky business: David had no insurance, and there was little money in the bank. A friend helped her to enroll in a business college, where she took a refresher course in bookkeeping, typing and shorthand. Roger Roscoe, manager at GWG (Great Western Garments) hired Dorothy, and she worked there on and off for thirteen years.

About a year after David's death, Roderick McPherson came into the picture.

Five years younger than Dorothy, Rod seemed happy and willing to take on the responsibility of two small children. Rod's father approved of the marriage, believing that Dorothy "had been through the mill and would make a better wife than a twenty-year-old single woman." Rod McPherson adopted the two children, and they all became McPhersons. From the beginning Rod proved himself a loving stepfather; he and young Gary "idolized each other," according to Dorothy. Dorothy and Rod's son Scott was born in January 1952, and the next year the family moved to the Yukon to a "big-paying job," at three hundred dollars a month. It seemed like a good move—until polio struck.

> The post-war epidemic of poliomyelitis, which for five years had been making its way west from Austral-Asia, reached Edmonton in the spring of 1953.
>
> It was as if this vibrant, optimistic city had been smitten by a medieval plague; it engendered the same fear and helplessness. Arbitrary and insidious, it struck all ages and conditions, sweeping its victims from buoyant health to paralysis and death within a week.
>
> Like war and like plague, it left its mark on three generations.[1]

Known in some areas as infantile paralysis, in the 1950s the disease poliomyelitis was still exacting a heavy toll in lives lost and limbs paralyzed—in adults as well as children. In 1954–55, health authorities launched a program to protect children in the Yukon against the feared disease. A public health nurse travelled to Watson Lake once a month, vaccinating children, beginning with the little ones, considered the most vulnerable, then progressing to older children as more vaccine became available.

"People were terrified of the disease," Betty George, a nurse at the University of Alberta Hospital in Edmonton, recalled. How was it transmitted? Through the air? By food contaminated with bacteria? No one knew. (Later the real culprit was found: polluted water.) In the early 1950s polio stalked the country during the summer months, striking at random. The *Edmonton Journal* published almost-daily reports of the devastating 1953 epidemic. Communities reacted by closing swimming pools and theatres. Playgrounds were deserted. Some city-dwellers took refuge in their summer cottages, trying—often in vain—to escape the scourge. Homes where some family member was known to have the disease were shunned, socially sealed off, as in the days of the Black Death that devastated Europe from 1347 to 1351.

• • • • •

FRANK ELLIOTT OF EDMONTON was one of many doctors alarmed with the ravages of the disease in 1953. "It was life-threatening and too often fatal, and its incidence reached epidemic proportions. We had never seen this before," he wrote.[2] On one November day Edmonton's isolation hospital was jammed with fifty-five patients, thirty-three of them on respirators. Five nurses were among the victims that year, and two died. One doctor was stricken and barely survived, another was left hemiplegic, and Frank Woodman, a physician from Westlock, Alberta, died.

In desperate moves to stop the contagion, health officials resorted to spraying DDT around and cleaning up all garbage and waste. The efforts were frantic and misdirected because no one really understood how the disease was spread.

But doctors did know something about the pathology of the disease. It was caused by a virus that attacked certain cells in the spinal cord

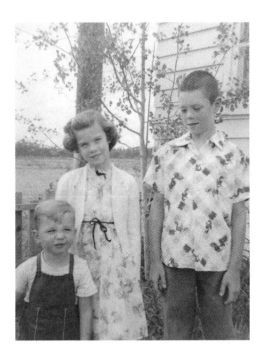

Gary, aged nine, and siblings Joanne and Scott McPherson at home in Swift River, a village in the Yukon in July, 1955.

responsible for the integrity and movement of muscles. The virus could also spread upwards to the brain and cause paralysis of the centres for swallowing, breathing and other vital functions.

Franklin Roosevelt, former American president and himself a polio survivor, created the National Foundation for Infantile Paralysis (now known as the March of Dimes), a private foundation devoted to funding research designed to eliminate the disease. Money raised by the March of Dimes supported a researcher working in the basement of an almost-empty isolation hospital in Pittsburgh. That researcher was Dr. Jonas Salk, professor in the Department of Bacteriology and Virology at the University of Pittsburgh. Salk was apparently not popular among his colleagues, but to millions he would become a hero.

Salk was building on the work of other men. John Enders of Harvard University had received the Nobel Prize in 1954 for isolating the polio virus. Jules Freund, of Belleview Hospital, New York, had developed a media suitable for vaccination. Salk learned how to grow the virus outside the body, then added killed polio virus to Freund's media in the hope that the vaccine would stimulate antibodies in the child and thus protect him or her against the disease. Salk received great help from Connaught Laboratories in Toronto: they were able to grow the polio virus in large quantities for him.

Salk then took the bold step of using the new vaccine to inject school-children in Pittsburgh, including his own. It was nail-biting time for him and his colleagues. But the vaccine worked: Salk measured antibody levels and found them sufficiently raised to protect a child against attacks by the polio virus.

History was made. On April 12, 1955, after a year of trials, the Salk vaccine was considered safe, and Salk was welcomed at the White House by President Dwight Eisenhower. In a few cases the vaccine failed because it didn't immunize against all types of the polio virus. Later, the Sabin vaccine was developed, using live but attenuated virus; put on the tongue in a lump of sugar, it proved to be almost one-hundred-percent reliable. By 1961, the incidence of polio in Canada and the United States had dropped by ninety-five percent.[3]

Salk was working on the vaccine in the 1940s, but it did not become generally available until the 1950s. Supplies were then gobbled up like gold. In 1954–55, schoolchildren in the Yukon aged seven and under, including Gary's sister Joanne, were vaccinated.

Nine-year-old Gary did not qualify for Salk's vaccine.

3 | Polio Strikes

IT WAS LIKE GETTING THE FLU, the way Marion "Beaver" Chomik, Gary's hospital roommate, described it.

In the fall of 1955, the McPherson family left the Yukon for a short holiday in Edmonton. The warm weather was over, and with it, the polio scare. Neither Rod nor Dorothy gave it a thought.

During the night of Saturday, October 1, the day before they were to return to the Yukon, nine-year-old Gary got sick. His family was staying with their friends John and Elsie Wilkins, whose son Rick was about Gary's age. Gary woke up that morning with a headache, nausea and a high fever. Rick dashed up to the kitchen from downstairs, where the boys slept in bunk-beds. Gary's mother hurried down.

Aware of some of the physical signs of polio, she asked Gary to put his chin on his chest. His neck was so stiff that he could hardly raise his head. He was rushed off to the isolation ward of the Royal Alexandra Hospital.

In a coma for the next ten days, Gary of course has no recollection of what happened to him. Within two days of his admission to hospital, he lost all movement in his limbs. More seriously, he stopped breathing and turned blue. Working at emergency speed, ward staff covered his face with a breathing mask and forced air into his lungs—a temporary

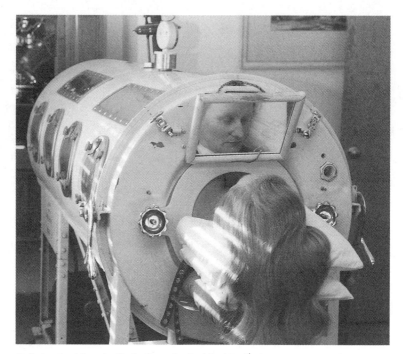

Polio patient Connie Clarke (now Packer) inside the iron lung. Connie Packer

measure. Then he was whisked into a Drinker-Collins iron lung, an airtight, elongated tank-like structure where the alternating positive and negative pressure would make up for his paralyzed breathing muscles. Only his head and neck remained outside.

Soon afterwards, he needed a tracheotomy (surgical opening in the windpipe) to facilitate the flow of air to and from his lungs, and to allow the suction of mucous secretions from his bronchial tubes. It was done for his benefit, but it took away his speech—he couldn't say a single word. The inability to tell anyone how he felt or what he needed was almost unbearable. "I felt bewildered, cut off and sometimes came close to panic," he recalled. Fortunately, if one of the staff held a finger over the opening in his windpipe, he could say a few words until his breath ran out. The tracheotomy (or "trake," as he called it) would be his companion for the next two years.

Gary's life-threatening illness jolted the McPherson family like an exploding bomb. Suddenly everything was called into question. There was no way they could go back to the Yukon, whatever the consequences. Rod could never desert the adopted boy whom he treated as his own son. So they stayed in Edmonton for all of October and part of November, travelling to the hospital at least twice a day. Then Rod made up his mind: he would go back to the Yukon and give up his job, then resettle in Edmonton with the family. While Gary's hold on life remained so precarious, Rod and Dorothy were determined to stay with him in this time of crisis.

On October 15, 1955, Gary was transferred along with other respiratory polio patients to Station 32, a special polio ward at the University of Alberta Hospital. They were escorted by Dr. Russell Taylor, director of the program that dealt with the 1953 polio epidemic which hit Edmonton so hard. It was no fun travelling in an ambulance without a siren, so Gary motioned to Dr. Taylor to turn the siren on. As they rolled through the streets of Edmonton with the siren wailing, cars, buses and trucks all moved over to let them pass. It was the one bright spot for the boy from the Yukon.

Skinny, freckle-faced Gary was the youngest patient in a room of ten people. The iron lungs filled the ward with swooshing and chuffing sounds like the noises in a busy laundromat on a Saturday afternoon. Patients on the polio ward came and went, many of them reaching the end of their earthly lives. For the survivors, every day was considered "a borrowed day." From the beginning Gary's parents were given no assurance that he would survive. "They gave us no hope at all," Dorothy remembers. Gary believes that a child today with his degree of disability would probably not survive; someone would have "pulled the plug."

Looking back, Dorothy McPherson shakes her head, almost in disbelief, over the turn of events. On October 15, 1955, it took only a few minutes in a fast-moving ambulance to get her son to the University Hospital. But the hospital stay turned out to last thirty-four years. Gary finally moved into his own home on October 19, 1989.

4 | When Life Hung in the Balance

"It was a terrible affliction for a kid," said Dr. Ted Aaron, one of the physicians caring for polio patients. "Gary was isolated in the iron lung and unable to move. He had to look in a mirror to see what was going on around him. He couldn't do a thing for himself, not a thing. On top of all that he couldn't breathe on his own. What could be worse?"

All the patients in the large room were, like Gary, "respiratory-dependent." Some were adults; others, teenagers just a few years older than him. All lived in a precarious state. Some time later Gary noticed that the ward had no clothes closets; he concluded that the planners had envisaged only short-term survivors.

The virulent attack of polio destroyed all movement in his arms and legs, and paralyzed his diaphragm, the most important muscle for breathing. Paralysis and wasting of his back muscles left him with severe scoliosis (curvature of the spine). When Gary regained a tiny amount of movement in his left hand over the next few months, he felt like he was "moving up into another grade." Eventually he recovered enough action in his left leg to enable him to propel his wheelchair backwards a few feet. His useless right hand lay at his side, palm up and completely inert.

Gary suspected that he probably wouldn't live very long, and that if he did live, he would never walk again and would likely be on a respirator for the rest of his life. Today he believes that being a child helped him to cope; he had not lived long enough to grasp the full significance of that prognosis. He often fantasized about walking again, but the disability never weighed heavily upon him. Even at this early stage, he started to think about what he could do rather than what he couldn't do. And he remained hopeful that some of the paralyzed muscles would eventually start to move again.

The harsh news seemed more cruel to Roderick and Dorothy McPherson. They gained some consolation in seeing their son holding on and making a slow recovery from the acute attack. But they had desperately hoped to see some return of movement in his paralyzed limbs. A letter they received from the doctor during a return trip to the Yukon effectively killed that hope, stating, "This boy is crippled for life."

Rod in particular was devastated by the news. It bothered him to see a promising boy so terribly incapacitated, reduced to a state almost worse than death. But the parents resolved to stick with Gary through thick and thin. Gary remembers well those hospital visits when "they used to bring me some decent food." Joanne, Gary's sister, felt like she had lost a brother she could always count on. "It's very, very hard when you have your big brother taken away. It's very hard," she said.

As the ravages of the polio virus subsided, dangerous breathing problems took over. A ward with critically ill patients in close quarters set the stage for chest infections, and Gary was hit with a severe bout of pneumonia on more than one occasion and a collapsed lung on another. But the inability to breathe on his own frightened him most, far more than the paralysis of his arms and legs. During the short periods when he was taken out of the iron lung, he struggled in vain for the breath that would not come. It filled him with a cold fear and showed up in blue fingertips. "In terms of low points in my life," he said, many years later, "there was nothing worse than not being able to breathe." To this day he remembers the loud sucking sounds and the irritating—sometimes agonizing—

discomfort when a nurse passed a catheter down into his bronchial tubes.

One night a complication developed that might have ended his life, had it not been for an alert young doctor racing to the emergency.

After the lights had been turned out, Gary was lying in the iron lung, trying to rest. Sleep was out of the question—he could feel himself getting weaker and weaker from lack of air. Thick mucous blocked his airway, and try as they might, the nurses could not suck it out through the tracheotomy opening. Gary panicked, feeling he would suffocate for sure.

"Can you come right away, Dr. Lakey!" an out-of-breath nurse cried, hammering on the door. Dr. Bill Lakey, then doing a year of research as part of his training in surgery, shared with a colleague a room not far from the polio ward. If any patient got into trouble during off-hours, the staff would run down the corridor and haul one of the young doctors out of bed.

Bill Lakey threw a white coat over his pyjamas and dashed down to the ward. He was appalled by the sight before him—a young boy who had turned blue. In the throes of hypoxic dementia (confusion from oxygen deprivation), his head rolled wildly from side to side; the rest of his body was motionless. Bill held his hand over the tracheotomy opening— no air was moving. He grabbed a catheter, shoved it down and tried to suck out a thick plug of mucous that he suspected was blocking Gary's airway. Nothing happened. He was desperate.

He suddenly realized the tracheotomy tube itself must be blocked, and "with great trepidation," he pulled it out. Almost immediately, Gary's blue lips turned pink and his head stopped rolling. The alert young doctor then inserted a new tube and tied it in place. He sucked out thick mucous lower down in Gary's bronchial tubes. After a few minutes of waiting to make sure his patient was out of trouble, he walked back to his room and returned to bed.

Forty-five years later, Gary remembers vividly the dramatic life-and-death episode. "I felt euphoric afterwards, just being able to breathe. It remains a low-high point for me, fixed forever in my mind." Gary maintains that Dr. Bill Lakey saved his life, but Bill is not so sure. He too remembers that emergency call during the night but, modest gentleman that he is, says that he was lucky to have been able to "yank out the plugged tube and put in a new one."

5 | **The Polio Ward**

A Unique Community

RON WILLSON started working as an orderly on the polio ward in January 1956, three months after Gary McPherson arrived. The first day on the job was pretty traumatic and bewildering. His head swam with all the strange sights and sounds. "Maybe I should have been frightened by it all, but there just wasn't time to be scared," he said. "There was work to be done, and it never ended. And the orderlies did most of the work."

Station 32 of the University Hospital housed thirty-five patients with polio. In Gary's room ten male patients, all more or less respiratory-dependent and needing iron lungs, lined both sides of a central corridor. Superimposed on the swooshing sounds of the iron lungs were the high-pitched sucks of tracheotomy tubes being cleared of mucous secretions. Periodically, sharp hisses from oxygen tank valves added to the madrigal of sounds. From the "hopper room" came even more discordant noises: metal clanging, bedpans being sterilized, flushing and gurgling. For each patient, the ear could—or rather, had to—adapt to this cacophony of aural stimuli, which thankfully tended to taper off a little at night. The nose, a master at accommodation, soon got used to the pungent smell of rubbing alcohol, soap of all scents, food and its variable aromas and, for want of better words, "bathroom smells."

Ron Willson and his co-workers found themselves facing formidable tasks, often feeling unqualified to be caring for so many critically ill patients. Ron had to keep his ear constantly attuned for the sounds of breathing problems in these voiceless patients with tracheotomies, frequently running to suck out gurgling mucous. Some patients learned to "click" loudly with their tongue when they needed help. Whenever a patient had to be removed from the iron lung for any length of time, they had to be "bagged." That meant forcing air into their lungs using a sort of balloon connected to a tight-fitting face mask. A few could breathe on their own for short periods; others were quite incapable of doing so.

Each iron lung had four portholes: one large and three small. Through these openings bedpans were passed, blood samples taken and patients bathed. When taken out of the lungs for changing of sheets and gowns, nearly all the patients had to be bagged.

Gary remembers the regimentation of the polio ward, with shift changes at 7:00 A.M., 3:00 P.M. and 11:00 P.M. Sometimes one staff person would feed breakfast to three patients at once. After breakfast came the routine of washing, bedpans and dressing. As a child, Gary was considered suitable to be bathed by one of the female staff, an arrangement he resented. "I wanted to be treated like an adult, even though I was a kid in an adult world." Some patients were taken on stretchers to physiotherapy. Visiting hours ended at 8:00 P.M., followed by lights-out.

One day, early in 1956, Gary's life took what he calls a great leap forward. With the staff, especially the doctors, encouraging him, he was moved temporarily from the iron lung to a flat bed, then connected to a chest respirator, a device that fitted the contours of his chest and was hooked up to a machine. He still needed assisted breathing and was not yet ready to be weaned off the apparatus. He then tried the rocking bed. A flat bed that can be tilted up and down to almost any angle, it assists breathing by using gravity to move the abdominal viscera up and down and indirectly draw air into the lungs. But the rocking bed made him seasick, and Gravol didn't help.

He will never forget the day he was lifted out and propped up in a wheelchair for a few minutes; being wheeled about was an incredibly freeing sensation. In due course he would get his own wheelchair, a blue one donated by the Canadian Legion. It would last him for fourteen years.

For most of the patients, the total dependency on others proved to be less of a sentence and more of a profound learning experience. But for some it was a painful lesson, and for a few a soul-destroying ordeal. It took Connie Clarke nearly two years to accept that she would never walk again. "I was terrible to everyone," she recalled. But she did learn, and with her sweet and charming personality she became years later the central figure for reunions of former polio patients. Gary was pretty good at sassing the nurses, but he too learned. Being a child with nineteen "mothers" all on his side, he tended to be forgiven a lot of things. "Oh, he was naughty all right," Connie said. "But he could flash a smile that would melt anyone's heart."

Ron Willson worked on the polio ward for eighteen months before reluctantly leaving. "I wouldn't have believed you could have so much fun at a job. It became my life," he said. "We did everything for them; we were their hands and feet." Ron developed a real skill at picking up the faintest clicking sounds and even reading the lips of tracheotomy patients. Like the rest of the staff of this remarkable ward, Ron saw his job as helping to salvage the disease-battered bodies of people whose minds and personalities remained healthy and wholesome.

. . . . .

OVER A PERIOD OF THREE YEARS, from 1955 to 1958, the polio patients on Station 32 grew into a remarkable community. They were a strange lot, many of them stricken with a monstrous disease and clinging to life by a fraying thread, yet full of zest. As the youngest, Gary had wonderful opportunities to learn lessons galore and to hear from his seniors everything they said, good and bad.

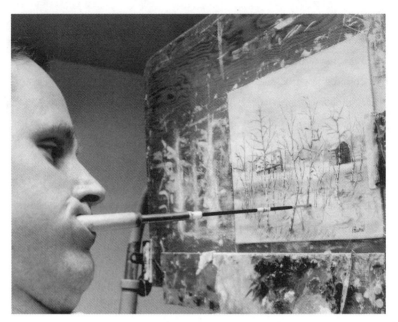

An undaunted artist, mouth-painter Henri Baril. Edmonton Journal

From the beginning he received special attention from the other patients in his room, even if he couldn't communicate with them. With the passage of time he could tolerate longer periods out of the iron lung, and with his tracheotomy tube plugged by a golf tee, he could pay more attention to his surroundings and talk to others. The mobility of a wheelchair did wonders for his interaction with others.

Togetherness was inevitable. Privacy was nonexistent: who could possibly hide anything?

Betty George was charge nurse for those years, and although Gary annoyed her—"Sometimes he made me so mad; he was lippy and rebellious"—she admired the overall morale of her patients. "They were like a big family." The nurses and orderlies became part of that family, and when patients were well enough for outings, they drove them to hockey games, lugging along chest respirators and breathing bags.

The ward became the patients' world. They could play cards with the help of an able-bodied person placing the cards in a rack with thin slots.

They could turn the pages of a book or magazine by holding a rubber-tipped stick with their mouths. A volunteer taught mouth-painting; two patients, Donna Graham and Henri Baril, became skilled at this art form.

The ward was like a special enclave in the great hospital, an enclave where hospital rules tended to get bent or ignored. Administrative nurses would simply stand at the door and call, "Is everything all right?" Whether deterred by all the iron lungs and respirators or by the knowledge that most patients were long-term, they rarely entered the ward or took any action. Or perhaps they saw nothing wrong with giving a few special privileges to the respiratory polio patients just barely hanging on to life.

The whole atmosphere could easily have been one of gloom and despair. Gary soon realized that people around him were dying, and for the first time he became aware of his own mortality. Yet despite the constant stream of life-threatening and irreversible illness, the ward remained a cheerful place, buoyant with high spirits and good humour. When Dr. Ted Aaron first looked in on it, he was surprised to find good-natured banter, joking and smart remarks bouncing from one side of the ward to another. As Gary remembers, a lot of the joking was "hospital humour that can be really gross" and it passed over his youthful head. But it was all part of a wonderful camaraderie.

No pets were allowed in the hospital, of course, but one day a friend or relative smuggled in a budgie. Allowed to fly freely around the room, the bright yellow bird would sometimes alight on one of the iron lungs and peer through the porthole to see what was going on. At other times, when a patient was being fed, it would perch right alongside in the hopes of getting a morsel or two. One day the nursing supervisor phoned up; she had heard about the budgie.

"The bird is kept in a cage, I trust," she said.

Betty George had answered the phone. She suddenly realized whose side she was on.

"Why, of course it is," she answered, crossing her fingers to cover up a small lie. At that moment the bird was doing circuits from one end of the ward to the other.

Betty George could cover up for the patients, but she was constantly on the *qui vive*, watching for anything going wrong. The iron lungs all operated from a bellows inside the tank that provided the changes in pressure to push air in and out; a small electric motor operated the bellows. A power failure, therefore, could be disastrous.

This fearsome event happened one evening when Betty was on duty. She dashed to the far end of the ward to activate the auxiliary power source, only to find that it wouldn't work. She put out a distress call to all the other wards for emergency help. Nurses and orderlies streamed through the door and took over manual operation of the bellows. Not one life was lost. Betty George called it "a miracle."

"The polio ward, in a sense, became my family," said Gary. At times his buddies on the ward seemed closer than members of his biological family, attentive though they certainly were to him. He admitted that "even though I must have been an irritation and a brat," he felt a love and a caring that kept him going. A group of five or six respiratory quadriplegics would, in time, become like brothers. If any of them felt low or discouraged, the others simply refused to let him get away with it, even if it meant hurling an insult or two.

6 | Young Gary

Growing and Learning

IT WAS LIKE NURTURING a stunted, withered plant. The polio virus had left Gary with four wasted limbs which lay on his bed, limp and immobile. His atrophied muscles would never regain their bulk and contour. Respiration, an essential function for human life that usually requires no conscious purpose, would for Gary henceforth be a dicey business requiring deliberate concentration and effort.

Fortunately, concentration and effort—and resolve—he did not lack. The first few trials at breathing outside of the iron lung were filled with fear, but he was determined to go on. More than two years passed before he could say farewell to the big metal tank and progress to assisted breathing with a chest respirator and sometimes the rocking bed.

One night during his sleep the tracheotomy tube fell out. Panicky, he called the nurse, who tried her utmost but could not reinsert the tube. Both nurse and patient decided to leave it out. No harm came from that decision, and the hole in his windpipe soon healed and Gary could talk again. The scar on the front of his neck is minimal, but as Gary said later, he has "scarred memories."

During physiotherapy, an important part of the rehabilitative care of polio patients, limbs were put through a range of movements in an attempt to avoid contractures (shortening or distortion) of muscles and ligaments. Patients were encouraged to try active movement of the few muscles that remained intact. Therapists soon determined that Gary's quadriceps (muscles on the front of his thighs) were capable of some movement, providing just enough strength in his left lower leg to shove his wheelchair backwards. He called these the only "decent-functioning muscles" in his legs. Gary considers himself fortunate to have recouped a little of the use of the fingers of his left hand, but the movements were uncoordinated and writing was—and remains—beyond his capabilities. Wanting desperately to learn to write, he took some training in mouth-writing, but found it impossible to combine it with breathing.

On Gary's first trip out of hospital, he was escorted with other patients to a concert by the great cowboy singer Gene Autry. His parents accompanied him, squeezing his breathing bag periodically to give him the air he needed. At the end of the performance, Gene Autry stood on the stage, ready to throw his white hat into the crowd as was his custom. But when he saw Gary below him in his wheelchair, he hopped down from the stage, took off his white Stetson and gently placed it on Gary's head. Dorothy still remembers the smile on Gene Autry's face, and the tears in his eyes. The next day he went up to the hospital's polio ward and auto-graphed the famous hat.

Later, the family brought Gary home every Sunday, but he had to be accompanied by a nurse. During his second year in hospital, he longed to go home to stay. Perhaps he was inspired by Bob Johnson, another young patient not quite so disabled, who left hospital on a short-term trial basis. The family did take Gary home for Christmas and cared for him as instructed by the staff. Gary's mother wanted to bring him home for good, despite the risks involved and the heavy round-the-clock responsibility that would fall upon her. Her husband had serious doubts and also felt that Gary would feel isolated. On the brink of indecision, they debated at length the pros and the cons. "When a little boy says he wants to come home, it's hard to say no," Dorothy said, but eventually they did say no, a decision that Gary accepted without disappointment or bitterness.

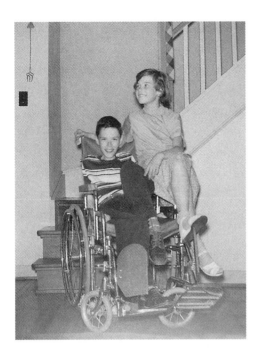

Gary and his sister Joanne visit on one of his short returns "home" from hospital.

It seemed abundantly clear that the hospital was destined to be Gary's "home." After a couple of years, the struggle for survival was no longer the top priority, replaced in rank by activities like schooling. In the Yukon Gary had reached grade five before polio cut off his education. Hospital staff or volunteers wheeled him down to a classroom on the children's ward, squeezing the breathing bag to supplement his own weak efforts. There were just ten kids in the class, all at different levels and hit with various afflictions.

Gary didn't much care for the class: he was afraid someone might suggest that he be transferred to the children's ward. He felt more secure on the adult ward with all the trained staff and respirators. One day during class-time a child suddenly fell to the floor, frothing at the mouth in an epileptic fit. It was a frightening experience for all the kids. Another time a child with leukemia started to bleed uncontrollably and had to be whisked away. Seeing these and other medical problems was a real learning experience for Gary, far more than the classroom teaching.

Later he took correspondence courses, getting help from volunteers turning pages and writing essays. Looking back, he has warm feelings of gratitude to the volunteers, mostly women, who devoted so many hours helping him to learn. But his heart wasn't in it. He didn't mind math but didn't care for literature, grammar or writing. Why bother with courses and studies when he would never live long enough to use any of it? But he did progress beyond the grade-five reading level, stimulated mainly by a growing passion for sports which spurred him to read newspapers. He would get someone to pin a page up on a line of string; after reading all he wanted on one page, he would then push his wheelchair around to read the other side.

He just couldn't get excited about formal or structured education. The hospital hired a part-time teacher for the children, but even he couldn't fan the feeble flame of Gary's desire. Maybe, just maybe, he could get inspired if he got into the public school system with all its social life and the competition he seemed to delight in. But the school authorities rejected his application for admission—the *coup de grâce* that killed any hopes or plans for a formal education. Looking back at that reversal years later, he could understand why no school in those days could have provided the assistance and accessibility he needed.

As a result, Gary never finished high school. He calls his schooling a hit-and-miss affair, partly due to his own apparent lack of interest. But a casual and indifferent approach to structured teaching did not mean an inability to learn, far from it. "Gary never bothered much with books," said Betty Fraser, a nursing aide on the polio ward from 1956 to 1959. "He just kept things in his head and never forgot anything he was taught."

Many people acquainted with the Gary McPherson of later years have asked, "What fanned the fire?" In light of spotty formal education, extreme physical disability and apparent lack of interest, how can you account for the intellectual giant of later years? Dr. Bob Steadward, presenter of Gary's honorary degree, said, "There aren't many university professors with the wisdom and smarts that Gary McPherson has."

Reg McClellan, an associate of Gary's in wheelchair basketball, has one explanation: "During his formative years, he was constantly surrounded by people with training and skills, people asking him questions and answering his." His mother, Dorothy, thinks that he became more focused in one direction as a result of his disability, and Rodney, his younger brother, believes he was a marvellous learner, gaining knowledge from everybody and everything. Bob Chelmick of Edmonton thinks that Gary developed his brain power "like a blind person develops the other senses to make up for the lack of sight." Walter Lawrence, a fellow quadriplegic, has a different idea: "Gary's suffering helped to hone his native talents."

Whatever the explanation, Gary's "victory" in the face of huge obstacles has been a source of vicarious pleasure for those involved in the early years of his career. Years later, Olga Warren, supervisor of the polio ward from 1956 to 1965, said it all with the words: "Gary, I'm so proud of you."

7 | A Brotherhood of Rogues

NEAR THE END OF 1958, the polio ward was moved to Station 67 of the University Hospital. This would be Gary's home for the next fifteen years.

Gary was now a teenager, one of a half-dozen young fellows all within six or seven years of each other. A close network of respiratory buddies in precarious health, they became known as "the boys," forming a brotherhood so tightly bonded that their respective families got involved with the care and support of any of the six needing help. In the cosmology of the polio ward, this brotherhood was venerated above all else.

In close proximity, they could scarcely avoid irritating and annoying each other. They argued and hurled salvos of abuse and insults, but underneath lay a oneness that each treasured. "I grew to love them deeply," Gary said. They did things as a group and supported one another from any perceived "assault" from whatever source, including hospital administration.

Arnie Stebner, about the same age as Gary, came over from the Edmonton General Hospital in 1957. A quadriplegic like the others, he retained enough function in his right arm to be able to write. Arnie's family "adopted" the boys and considered them all sons. They often invited them to their home in town and to their cottage at Pigeon Lake,

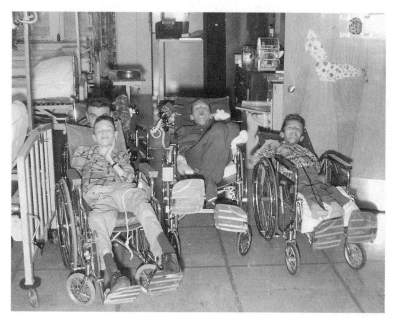

"The boys": the four Polio ward respiratory buddies, in 1959. From left to right, Gary McPherson, Henri Baril (half hidden), Clayton May and Arnie Stebner.

not far from Edmonton. On a Sunday afternoon his mother sometimes shared a Bible story or lesson with Arnie, and the others would listen in.

Henri Baril, a bright, congenial French-Canadian several years older than Gary, contracted polio in 1954 and ended up totally disabled, even worse off than Gary. He became a proficient frog-breather to assist his weakened respiratory muscles; not for a couple of years would Gary learn and perfect this technique. Gary chuckled while saying that he received his sex education from Henri, who got his in turn from the orderlies. A gifted mouth-painter, Henri sold his work to a foot- and mouth-artists' association that published Christmas cards.

Marion Chomik, or "Beaver," had front teeth which reminded his buddies of Canada's national emblem. Living in Viking, Alberta, he got polio in 1960 when he was about twelve years old. He and Gary became the best of friends and lived as roommates in adjacent beds for many years.

Beaver was also a quadriplegic, but he fortunately retained considerable movement in his right arm and right leg.

Bob Johnson from Big Valley, Alberta, was the entrepreneur, the go-getter of the group. A tall redheaded boy, he was outside the age range of the others, being thirteen years older than Gary. He was more or less the organizer and the "boss." At one time Bob's family lived in an apartment next door to the McPhersons. His degree of paralysis was a little less than Gary's: he could sit upright, breathe fairly easily and write with difficulty. His brother Doug described Bob as "fiercely independent" and wondered if some of that rubbed off on Gary.

Sandy Burgess broke his neck in a diving accident and became totally paralyzed from the neck down. A six-footer who got injured in Halifax, he was the only non-polio member of the group. By the time he reached Station 67, he had progressed beyond the iron lung and tracheotomy stage. Gary remembers him as having "a great disposition and amazing motivation." He completed high school and eventually went to university, doing all the writing and typing with his mouth. Betty George believes Sandy was "a tremendous inspiration to Gary, showing what he could accomplish."

Clayton May came to the ward from the General Hospital with Arnie. A couple of years older than Arnie and Gary, he was totally paralyzed below the neck from polio. Like Arnie, he had acquired some skill with frog-breathing, but he used an iron lung to sleep at night. Clayton was thoughtful and wise, a deep thinker and an engaging conversationalist. If anyone was a mentor to Gary, it was Clayton.

When Lorraine Habekost first landed on the polio ward as a nursing aide in 1962, she shook her head, wondering what kind of "circus freaks" lived attached to all the rocking beds and respirators and other devices. She soon found out what a spunky lot they were. Far from being inert, they seemed to keep the place hopping, even if they had little physical movement themselves. Her job was bedside nursing, including changing sheets, bathing, suctioning, feeding and giving tracheotomy care.

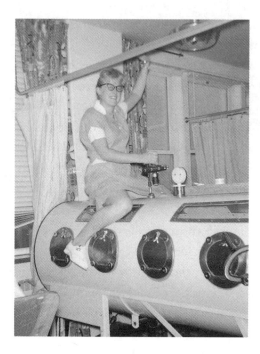

At work and play, nursing aide Lorraine Habekost astride an iron lung.

She got to know each one of "the boys" and considered them part of her family. She and other staff members helped with their parties, and they weren't "pity parties" either, far from it. The staff would bring in lots of food, and Lorraine admitted, "the booze somehow got in too." A few times they brought in a three-piece band, and there was singing and dancing. It was quite a sight to see nurses and nursing aides propelling the patients in wheelchairs around the dance floor.

Of course there were sad times, and many tears. Olga Warren was supervisor of the polio ward when a six-year-old girl, Jeanie Mark, was admitted, unable to breathe. For Olga, the sight of a polio-stricken child on a stretcher was far from unfamiliar, but this time it was almost too much. Later that day, with sobs and sighs she related her feelings to her brother and moaned, "If we have a good God, why can't Jeanie breathe?" Peter told her, "You can never help Jeanie, or anybody, if you walk around with a long face. You've got to go there and smile, even if it kills you." But sometimes, Lorraine said, it was impossible to smile. When someone died, "it was like losing a member of the family. The staff too would be around the corner, wiping their eyes."

Through the joys and stormy trials and the sadness, this rather unique "family" closed ranks to support each other; the combination of caring and courage often touched the lives of outsiders. Years before being elevated to the position of judge, Don Buchanan became a friend of the boys when he hobbled down to the ward on crutches while recovering on a nearby ward from an orthopedic operation. He called them "heroic friends."

Some years later he brought to the polio ward a secretary at a law firm, a young woman in the depths of despair and depression. "We sat down by Clayton's bedside, drank a glass of wine together, listened to Clayton's records and laughed together," Don said. That ended her depression. "She said that visit changed her there and then—just seeing somebody in that terrible disabled state and yet so happy and uncomplaining."

The boys lived in mere shells of bodies, but they faced all the puzzlement and quandaries of adolescence. Girls were on their minds much of the time, and they often lusted to touch them. Some days their hormones seemed to be running wild, stimulated by a well-rounded bosom or a shapely leg. Gary admits that during his teenage years, he "fell in love frequently with one of the beautiful young volunteers or student nurses" and didn't know how to express himself. "The more deprived you are, the more you think about it," he said. It tended to become an obsession—and a frustration. Sexuality grew into an even greater frustration when the mother of one of his buddies told him outright that the Bible made it clear that it was wrong to look at a woman with lust in your eyes. Being unable to reconcile his powerful inner feelings with the teachings of the Bible made him uncomfortable.

For a time Gary put the church aside, but not spirituality. Unlike able-bodied teenagers, he was acutely aware of his own mortality, and every time a death occurred on the ward—and death seemed to be always hovering nearby—that awareness was reinforced. But he found no answers, although he did resolve to one day "improve myself as a person for this life and the next."

Years later he could confidently assert that "one of the strongest tools you can have in life is faith, faith in yourself, in God and in other people. Without faith, you can't go anywhere."

8 | The Frog-Breather

LEARNING HOW TO FROG-BREATHE was a life-defining moment for Gary, a turning point that grew into a kind of epiphany. Conferring on him an independence and a freedom comparable to that provided by his beloved blue wheelchair, it was the culmination of a long battle against the forces hostile to respiration, so to speak.

After escaping from the iron lung, he progressed to the vertigo-causing rocking bed and thence to the chest respirator, or cuirass. Like a turtle shell strapped to his chest, it was connected to a machine that produced negative pressure and then released, thereby drawing air into and out of his lungs. The cuirass helped many patients, but Gary was so thin and bony and his back so twisted with scoliosis that it could not be made to fit. It didn't really help much. A custom-made respirator worked for a few years, but he often had to return to the iron lung at night to get proper oxygenation. Then he progressed to a Monaghan positive pressure respirator hooked up to a mouthpiece, which afforded him good ventilation at night.

Using neck muscles and the little that remained of his diaphragm, he could breathe on his own for a couple of hours before exhaustion and anoxia (lack of oxygen) set in and he had to go back to the respirator. But

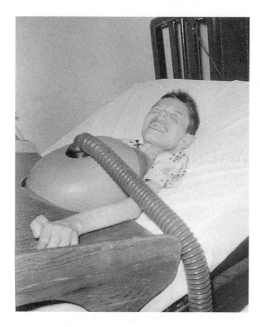

Gary breathing with the help of a chest respirator or "cuirass."

he was determined to breathe without any apparatus, no matter what it took in effort and hours of persistence.

Frog-breathing (or more technically, glossopharyngeal breathing) was the key that a couple of Gary's fellow polio survivors had mastered. They learned to consciously gulp in a breath of air, then contract the muscles of the tongue (glossa) and throat (pharynx) to pump air down into the lungs. Inflating the cheeks like a frog is not necessary. As Gary describes it, you hold your breath and add to it with gulps of air. Having learned the skill, a patient can live and work independently during the day, away from a respirator or any other equipment.

Henri Baril, one of the boys who had acquired much skill at mouth-painting, was fortunate enough to "stumble across it" one day when he was out of the iron lung. Martin Pudar from Sangudo, Alberta, was another patient who somehow acquired the technique without much effort.

But for Gary, it was a different matter. He took instruction from Bea Martin, a physiotherapist who had gained experience in teaching the technique in a big polio ward at Rancho Los Amigos, California, near Los

Angeles. While Gary tried frog-breathing, she clipped something like a clothes-peg on his nose, then held a feather in front of his mouth to determine whether he was actually moving any air in and out. Most times she just stood back and shook her head. The feather hardly fluttered. Gary got pretty discouraged. "I just couldn't learn, no matter who tried to teach me."

Then one day in 1962 it came—out of the blue, he said. But that wasn't quite true: he had been working at it on his own for many long months. He was sitting out by the nursing station and suddenly found himself taking good breaths, using the technique that Bea Martin had been trying to drill into him. It was a special day for him, his friends and his family; it meant that Gary could actually start thinking about the future that heretofore had been highly uncertain, if not out of reach.

Lorraine Habekost remembers that it wasn't long before Gary was rolling his wheelchair up to the beds of others who were trying to learn frog-breathing. "He was very patient with them, remembering how long it took him to learn," she said. Years later, in collaboration with the respiratory therapy department of the Aberhart Hospital, Gary made a video that described the method and the use of frog-breathing. This video was presented at a worldwide polio conference in St. Louis, Missouri, in 1983.[1]

Frog-breathing changed Gary's life. In years to come he would gain renown as a much-in-demand public speaker. Without frog-breathing, he could never have given the outstanding address at the university convocation in 1995, an address that rated a standing ovation by the thousands in attendance.

Darlene Steljes, formerly a respiratory therapist, is not ordinarily given to making sweeping statements, but she is convinced that Gary is one of the longest-living mouth-ventilated people in the world.

9 | Outings Far from the Polio Ward

THE WELL-USED YELLOW 1954 TRAVELLALL VAN was far from fancy, but "it gave us a new lease on life," Gary said. "We felt liberated; we went everywhere in it." The van, a gift from Arnie's uncle who worked for Leduc Construction, could hold five boys in their wheelchairs, but there were no seat-belts and no tie-downs. The wheelchairs were rolled up an old wooden ramp, jammed in, and the door slammed tight; the tighter the fit, the better. Bob Johnson wrote an article about the beloved canary-coloured van in *The Caliper* under the headline "Have Old Yeller, Will Travel."[1]

With their portable respirators onboard, they did travel, but not without some anxious moments. Once the old van spluttered to a halt on Jasper Avenue, Edmonton's main street, the last drops of gas dripping from the tank onto the pavement. Another time they took it to Calgary to see the annual Labour Day football game between the Edmonton Eskimos and the Calgary Stampeders. It was a six-hour trip, but Gary figures they were lucky to get there at all. They had barely reached Leduc when the front end of the old van was seized with paroxysms of vibration. It felt like they were riding on a jackhammer. They pulled over to the closest service station, where the van was hoisted high in the air. Suddenly a

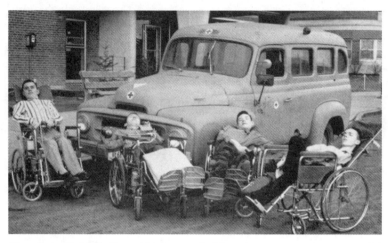

"June is bustin' out all over! And respos in Edmonton are eager to get out and enjoy it." Writer Bob Johnston featured buddies Marion Chomik, Arnie Stebner, Gary McPherson, and Clayton May posing in front of the "Old Yeller" van.
The Caliper

front wheel fell off and landed on the concrete floor. Someone had forgotten to tighten the bolts, and they had sheared off.

Later the generous Stebner family presented their polio-survivor friends with a red 1964 Ford Econoline van, which lacked the flaws and weaknesses of Old Yeller. It didn't have a hydraulic lift (a luxury that would come later), but it did carry strong, back-loaded aluminum ramps. The boys used the van to go everywhere. The Stebners paid for gas, insurance and operating costs; the boys had only to recruit the drivers, and they were available in abundance.

"Being able to travel around was good for us all in terms of independence and freedom," Gary said. "The Stebners wanted primarily to help Arnie, but their kindness included us all."

Staff and volunteers drove the Respos (respiratory polios), as they called themselves, around town with a nonchalance that almost defied belief. Despite some problems and difficulties, they never lost a patient. Sometimes in a restaurant when a tracheotomy tube needed suctioning, the escort would look around for an electrical outlet, plug in the portable suction machine and calmly proceed to do the job. For the other patrons the procedure caused some alarm, soon dispelled by the laughing and joking that followed.

Ron Fortin, an orderly on Station 67, barely weathered a "beads of sweat on the forehead" episode while escorting a respirator-assisted patient to a conference for mouth-painters. He had loaded the portable respirator into the backseat of a taxi, where it was connected to the car's battery, and was lifting the patient into the taxi when the inner part of his tracheotomy tube fell out. Ron laid the patient flat on the roadside and, working at top speed, managed to replace the part. He lugged the patient back into the taxi, then proceeded to make a second mistake: he jammed the hood of the taxi down onto one of the battery connections and short-circuited the battery. Smoke and acrid fumes belched forth alarmingly. But Ron was master of the situation: he bagged the patient to give him air, dug in his pocket for money to get a new battery for the taxi driver, and they were soon off to the conference, none the worse for wear.

Of all the staff who worked on Stations 32 and 67, Lorraine Habekost knew the polio patients best and loved them most. During her thirty-two years as a nursing aide on the wards, she saw them at their best and their worst. She grieved when they suffered, and at other times exulted and laughed along with them. When her baby was born, the patients rejoiced as if they were her own kin. In later years her child became a respiratory therapist "because of Gary's influence," she said.

Lorraine and her husband Norman often invited Gary and one or more of his polio-survivor friends to their cottage at a lake near St. Paul, Alberta, where Little Tana would observe her mother giving Gary the chest physiotherapy he needed every morning. One weekend Clayton, Gary and friends decided to roast a pig for the occasion.

In his usual methodical manner, Clayton had a friend borrow a book from the library to be sure the job would be done right. He carefully read the instructions, then got the able-bodied people to dig a deep hole and shovel in plenty of smouldering hot coals. Then they wrapped burlap and wet newspapers around the pig, dropped it into the pit and placed hot rocks around it. Everyone suggested it should then be covered with a layer of soil, but Clayton said it wasn't necessary. He knew best. Just wet a tarp and cover it lightly, he said.

Everyone disappeared into the cottage for a while, licking their lips in anticipation of tasty roast pork. In due course, Norman went out to inspect the roast.

"The pig's gone," he hollered. Everyone scurried out to the pit, wheelchairs and all. There was no pig to be seen, only a few charred coals. It had been effectively cremated. They all sat back and laughed. Clayton apologized and said that next time he would consult a different book.

10 | The Allure of Sports

From Cheering to Coaching

THE BOYS COULD ONLY DREAM about hitting a home run or stickhandling around the defence and firing a shot on goal. But nothing stopped them from being spectators, and to a man, they joined the ranks of enthusiastic sports fans. Gary loved sports and rarely missed reading the sports pages in the *Edmonton Journal*. The big TV set on the ward allowed them to watch hockey and football games, cheering and hollering as if they were there in the stands.

Dwayne Doberthein, one of the first and most consistent drivers willing to take the boys to football and hockey games, lived in the same apartment block as Bob Johnson's family and through Bob got to meet Arnie, Henri, Gary and the others. Dwayne had never hauled wheelchairs around or loaded them into a vehicle, but he soon learned, starting by escorting them to football games. Usually Gary had a respirator strapped to his chest. Then Dwayne took them to hockey games, first to see the Oil Kings play at the old Edmonton Gardens stadium and later to games featuring the Oilers. In no time Dwayne found himself overlooking the disabilities as the boys became his friends. "I just couldn't do enough for those guys," he said.

Sometimes it was a risky business watching Edmonton Eskimos football games at Clarke Stadium. Fans using wheelchairs had to sit at the bottom of the stadium, where they were often at the mercy of disgruntled fans throwing bottles and other debris from higher up. Seating facilities for the disabled improved greatly in the new Commonwealth Stadium. Young Gary McPherson had a hand in upgrading the space set aside for wheelchairs at the Edmonton Gardens, lobbying the Edmonton Exhibition Association to build a decent platform for them. His efforts were eventually successful, and the association provided a concrete platform. This was probably the first of many lobbying efforts to come.

Ernie Daigle never anticipated doing such a thing when he first started cutting the hair of the polio patients in 1957, but he ended up driving them to Eskimos football games for almost six years. After arriving at the stadium, he would roll out the wheelchairs, line them up in front of the football field and then watch the game with them. Sometimes he invited them to his home afterwards. "It was good for my kids to see guys so full of life," he said.

The outings to football and hockey games proved to be more than just entertainment for Gary. By shrewd observation along with some contact with managers and players, he learned much about team sports: how coaches treated players, what motivated players, what made for a winning team. As a "wheelchair kid," he was fortunate enough to get into the dressing rooms of some of the professional teams. The athletes were invariably willing to talk to him. Edmonton was on its way to becoming "The City of Champions," endowed with outstanding teams and athletes. Gary met and talked with some of the great athletes such as Jackie Parker, Warren Moon and Wayne Gretzky.

Unaware of it, he was being groomed for the time when he would be a coach and a manager himself, building a reputation that would elevate him all the way to the Sports Hall of Fame.

Another sport became a passion for the notorious group of six— horse-racing. It started when Don Buchanan, a serious devotee of the "Sport of Kings," first visited the polio ward, where he became a good friend of Clayton. After Don had recovered from his broken leg, he took

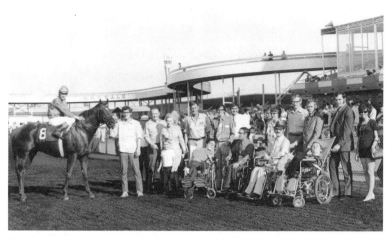

On August 10, 1971, "the boys," their family and friends cheered on Bob and Clayton's horse at Edmonton's Northlands Park. Northlands Park

the boys early in the morning down to the racetrack, where they admired the sleek horses, fed them sugar lumps and then watched the jockeys doing practice circuits. That sparked their interest, and when the racing season was on, they wanted to go down to the track almost every day. Those who couldn't go would get one of the others to place a bet for them. It became a serious business, and in due course Clayton and Bob, both farm boys originally, bought a horse. Unfortunately, it didn't perform as well as they hoped.

One day at the track, Gary and Bob were sitting in their wheelchairs when a man walked up, saying he too was interested in thoroughbred horses. They talked about affairs at the track, then he asked where they came from and why they were in wheelchairs. The man, who then introduced himself as Don Getty, was to become a lifelong friend of Gary.

Sports of all kinds caught Gary's attention, but it was slow-pitch softball that moved him a few years later from cheering to coaching.

· · · · ·

"Hey, you! Do you play ball?"

Janet Ross was running down the hall of the Aberhart Hospital, where she worked as a dietary aide in the kitchen. She stopped, turned around and saw a weird-looking, skinny fellow in a wheelchair. He smiled at her and repeated the question.

"Why, yes," said Janet. "In fact, I've been playing ball since I was a kid."

"Come and join our team. We have great times."

That was sixteen-year-old Janet's introduction to the mixed slow-pitch ball team of able-bodied players that operated out of the Aberhart Hospital. Gary McPherson coached the team. Soon she was knocking out flies and practising with the team, which went by the name of the Bad News AIRS (Aberhart Independent Recreation Society). The team began playing in a hospital league of staff, friends and relatives playing just for recreation, but soon expanded "because there wasn't enough competition." Initially Gary had the job of general manager, which included finding players to build up a team; later, he became coach. During the course of eighteen active years, the Bad News AIRS developed into a formidable team, twice winning league titles in the Edmonton Mixed Slow-pitch Association.

As soon as the snow melted in the spring, Gary was on the phone, calling for practices to begin. When the season began in earnest, they played twice a week and competed in a tournament on alternate weekends. Competition was keen, and as Gary Ogletree remembered, "some of the players were pretty hot-blooded."

Valerie Kamitomo, who had been playing the game as a pitcher from the age of twelve, joined the Aberhart team after graduation from nursing school. "But I didn't get to do much," she said, "because they were so good." For two years she sat by the coach, keeping score. By the time she got to play, she had learned the tactics and strategies of the game. Later she would become a very important person in the coach's life.

How did Gary ever get to be a coach? For that matter, how did he ever learn how to coach? He hadn't swung a bat or thrown a ball since he was a boy of nine. Bob Steadward attributed Gary's abilities to his shrewd powers of observation and perception. "He has an uncanny ability to absorb whatever is going on in front of him," he said. Peter Eriksson, formerly a wheelchair basketball coach in Sweden, says you don't need to have been a participant in order to coach effectively. Gary understood the strategies used by a winning team, and he put them to work. He utilized his players effectively, being able to analyze opponents' strengths and weaknesses, and unafraid to ask for input from his players. Often he would use one of the better players on the team as a role model for teaching others.

And he was a firm believer in visualization, the process of imagining and seeing situations or problems turning out the way you would like them to. Believing in Albert Einstein's claim that "Imagination is more important than knowledge," Gary told the players to visualize themselves hitting a home run or catching a fly in deep centre field. He encouraged them to visualize winning too, though not to the extent of allowing desire to interfere with enjoyment of the game.

The "people skills" acquired throughout his years in hospital, plus all the learning gleaned during his time with the Jaycees, stood him in good stead with the ball players. If someone dropped a fly, he or she would not receive a torrent of abuse from an inflamed coach, but rather a gentle urge to do better next time. (Team member Brian Riley wondered if Gary's weak breathing muscles kept him from hollering.) "He was good at encouraging people and building them up, focusing on their strengths," Janet said. But if the player dropped flies one after another, he or she might be banished to the bench for a while.

Gary was no softie. One male member of the team, a real heavy hitter and pressure-player, blew up during one game and threw a tantrum, threatening everyone around him and eventually getting ejected from the game by the umpire. Gary quietly called him aside to "soothe the beast" in him, cooled him down and reminded him that the team valued him, but only if he played the game in a civil manner. Others were amazed to see how a seething firebrand could be disciplined by a paralyzed man in a wheelchair.

The league required that each team have no fewer than three girls, a rule considered by some players to be a nuisance regulation. The AIRS had some strong female players, including Val Kamitomo and Adrienne Riley, both pitchers. Those two got lots of playing time; during one tournament Adrienne pitched five games in one day. While not requiring the energy of fastball, pitching for slow-pitch requires skill and concentration, something the average spectator does not appreciate. "A good pitcher can control the game," said Carlene Brenneis, who played second base. Gary understood the pressures under which a pitcher operates. Once, after Val had pitched three balls with no strikes, she just barely heard Gary's whisper, "Come on, Val. We're with you."

"Who's your coach?" hollered one member of the opposing team before the start of a game one day in Edmonton. "They would throw a quick look at Gary in his wheelchair, curl up their lips as if thinking, 'Boy, this team will be a pushover,' and snicker among themselves," recalled Lorraine Habekost, who also pitched for the AIRS. They got fooled many times. The frail-looking coach not only knew the game but was highly competitive. And if need be, he could baby-sit at the same time. Brian and Adrienne Riley sometimes brought two-year-old Jason along and left him in his stroller while they were playing. Gary had just enough strength in his left leg to rock the stroller to keep Jason from crying and lull him to sleep.

Carlene, an experienced player who worked with Val at the Cross Cancer Institute, joined the team along with her husband, Gary Ogletree. Neither one was concerned about Gary's disability, quickly learning that his understanding of the game was "tremendous." Gary (the player) played in the outfield, and before the start of one inning, he got a call from Gary (the coach) to shift his position to the right because the batter usually hit to that position. Somewhat doubtful, he did shift to the right. Sure enough, the batter hit the ball "right into my lap."

"We may not have had the best players," said Gary Ogletree, "but as a team we had some quality, hard to define, that allowed us to have fun together, and often win."

Janet has vivid memories of her first tournament with the AIRS team, when they competed one Canada Day weekend at St. Paul. It was stifling hot, dusty and decidedly unfriendly. "Everyone was cheering for our opposition." The AIRS were definitely the underdogs, but being "city slickers," they rated nothing but hisses and boos from the partisan crowd. "But that made us try all the harder," Janet said. The pressure was intense. Gary and his team made it through to the final game, sunburnt and exhausted. They came from behind to win the game, playing, Janet said, "with our hearts more than anything else."

They won the tournament and with it, a trophy and a lump sum of prize money. The *St. Paul Journal* published a front-page photo of the team standing around their coach's wheelchair, with a player holding up the trophy for him.[1]

Ron Minor, one of Canada's most skillful wheelchair athletes in his day, made an effort to see a couple of games featuring the Bad News AIRS team. "If you can manage people, they will play their hearts out for you," he said afterwards. "Gary inspired his players, but mostly because he befriended them first."

For Gary Ogletree and Carlene Brenneis, Gary represented a good role model for their kids as someone who did amazing things despite the odds stacked against him.

Said Carlene, "His commitment and total involvement with the slow-pitch team reflected his philosophy of life."

11 | Entrepreneurs and Innovators

"WE MAY BE DISABLED, BUT WE'RE NOT SICK," said the feisty and irrepressible residents—they no longer considered themselves patients—of Station 67. They somehow seemed to dissociate themselves from their physical state. For the Respos, the ward where they had lived for years was also their "turf." Others needed to be reminded of that, including hospital administration. Darlene Steljes found them "pretty abrasive" when she first arrived on the ward as a student in respiratory therapy. But she retaliated with a few sharp comments of her own and soon became their friend. "I was simply amazed by those polio patients," she said.

Few would deny the true grit and courage of those patients, but a casual observer could detect in an instant that they were blessed with wonderful allies in the nurses, therapists and orderlies, as well as the many volunteers. Olga Warren, who took over as ward supervisor in 1956, was known as "Mother" to Clayton, Arnie and Gary. "Our staff was unique. We were a family that worked together and played together," Betty Fraser said. "If any of us felt worried or grumpy when we left home in the morning, we tried to leave our feelings at the door of the ward. There was no way we would allow our personal problems to interfere with our work."

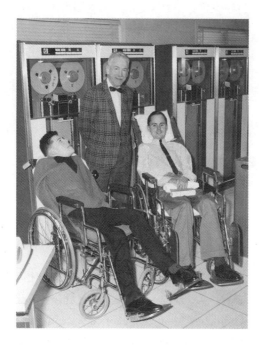

*Innovative entrepeneurs
Gary McPherson and
Henri Baril begin a
course in computer
programming under the
supervision of Dr. Don
Scott, dean of computing
science at the University
of Alberta.*

The University of Alberta Hospital

Whether or not they had earned their autonomy, they took it, seizing control of their lives and launching forth. Their bodies might have been imprisoned, but their minds were free to fly, even soar. Ideas, schemes, strategies and projects filled the air, then multiplied as they bounced from one Respo to another.

One venture got off the ground when Dr. Don Scott, dean of computing science at the university and chairman of the Canadian Paraplegic Association, heard about the enterprising six boys and offered to arrange a course on computer programming as a pilot project. Dr. Scott, himself a polio survivor with a disabled arm, sent over an attractive young instructor named Wanda Payne, who had no trouble keeping the attention of her students. Over the course of a few months of twice-weekly sessions, Wanda taught basic programming skills, including key punching and data entry. She gained their respect not only as a teacher but also as a woman of courage; she had been diagnosed with leukemia and was fully aware that her life would be short.

Computers were primitive in those days, Beaver recalled, and it didn't take the class long to learn. After they had completed the course, the university provided the boys with piecemeal work for which they were paid. Then another idea surfaced: why not start their own computer programming company? With Gary and Clayton pushing hard, they launched Pro-Data Services, with Bob Johnson as business manager and Beaver in charge of marketing. They did work for the university as well as for the hospital and a few business firms.

Demands for their services grew, so they hired a couple of students to work for them on a grant, using an empty room in the hospital. Eventually they moved into an apartment complex across the street and then into a downtown office. At one time they had a staff of twenty-seven, including some programmers imported from Britain. After the company grew into "a reputable company known for its quality work," Gary's part in its operation diminished as he got interested in other things.

After ten years the company closed its doors. Of the six boys, Beaver gained the most from the training and experience, and he eventually served as a consultant for Canadian Utilities before getting a permanent job with that firm. The company's demise was undoubtedly precipitated by the death of Bob Johnson, the third of the group to lose his life. Redheaded Bob was the business head and driving force of the company. He died from brain damage caused by anoxia when he passed out. According to Gary, "the impact of his dependency on alcohol had huge ramifications... for his family, friends and business colleagues."

About this time the boys embarked upon an activity that would "open up a whole new world for us." They became amateur radio operators. The seed was sown when Gary read an article about amateur radio in the *Toomey J. Gazette*, an international publication for and about polio survivors. The idea of conversing by radio with people all over the world piqued Gary's interest, but he didn't know how to proceed. Dr. Frank Haley, an anaesthetist at the University Hospital, possessed the *savoir-faire* to bring their dreams to reality.

Dr. Haley had a special interest in pulmonary function and the use of ventilators and other devices for assisted respiration. Pursuing that interest, he dropped in to the polio ward quite often and got to know the patients who were being weaned off rocking beds and cuirasses. When someone mentioned their interest in radio, he perked up his ears. He owned a ham radio set, having acquired his licence two years earlier in Saskatoon. He offered to help them set up their own station and immediately got four willing students to learn the ropes: Arnie, Clayton, Gary and Beaver. They would have to pass a technical exam and learn Morse code, at that time a requirement for ham radio operators.

Dr. Haley recruited some of his radio friends to come to the hospital and teach the boys how to receive and send the *dit-dah-dit* messages. Gary had slight movement of his left thumb and index finger, and he learned to send the code with the help of a custom-made key. Clayton had no such movement, but he could click with his jaw. Frank Haley asked a dentist friend to make a dental rim that would fit on his teeth, embedded in which was a microswitch hooked up to a transmitter. By clenching his teeth for short or longer periods, Clayton could make a *dit* or a *dah*.

But learning Morse code was just a start. They had to be able to send or receive twelve words a minute, and after a year of using Morse on the radio, they could qualify to use a microphone. To get their own station, they also had to pass an exam on the theory and practical aspects of radio; with the help of a volunteer who wrote down their answers, they passed with ease. After they had qualified, Dr. Olie Rostrup, an orthopedic surgeon at the hospital and the Canadian Legion, contributed most of the money for a transceiver able to transmit or receive. Then they applied for and got their licence and joined the Northern Alberta Radio Club.

Frank Haley somehow persuaded hospital administration to allow him to set up an antenna on the roof, with wires connected to the radio and a directional beam that could be rotated through cables running down to the ward. On that first day Frank and his small coterie of polio-

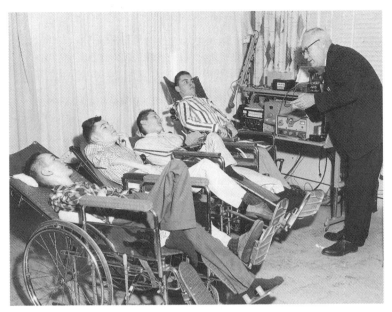

Instructor Bob Moore teaching the intricacies of ham radio operation to Clayton May, Gary McPherson, Arnie Stebner and Marion "Beaver" Chomik, from left to right.

survivor fans talked to a farmer in Saskatchewan and someone from Saudi Arabia.

The apparatus was set up near an outside wall for easy access to the wiring, quite close to Gary's bed. With a little help from the staff and the less disabled and the call signal VE6RD (RD for "respiratory-dependent"), they developed buddies across North America, many of them in institutions or shut in their own homes. One station called "The Handicappers" always welcomed them. Eventually they were speaking to people all over the world, some of whom later visited them on the ward during a trip to Edmonton.

Frank Haley called himself "the contact man" for the would-be radio operators, and although many contributed to the project in various ways, he was undoubtedly the key figure. Although initially he wondered "how wise it was to try to help those fellows and even to keep them alive when they were so severely handicapped," he soon dispelled those ideas.

While enjoying the ease of communication by radio, they had no inkling that their own little set with the hospital-rooftop antenna would ever serve a practical purpose, let alone one of crucial importance.

In 1968, the first Canadian Wheelchair Games were slated to be held in Edmonton at the University of Alberta. In the weeks before the games, a mail strike seriously disrupted communications. Officials agonized over such concerns as processing entries, passing information about transportation and organizing events. Long distance phone calls were prohibitively expensive.

Thanks to a Vancouver ham radio operator who had established "Links Across Canada" with fellow operators, help was at hand. Every Saturday at 9:00 A.M. a cross-Canada hookup with Edmonton at the epicentre brought everyone together, much like a telephone conference call, connecting the committees working for the games in centres across the country. Arnie, Beaver and Gary operated the radio, and if need be, they called local people by phone to hear or receive radio messages. But usually the local organizers for the games came to the polio ward to be by the radio.

How important was the role of the amateur radio set to the success of wheelchair basketball's first national championships? Gerry Way, a member of the organizing committee, gave a clear answer: "Gary and his buddies did a super job. They saved the games."

Up to then Gary knew little about sports for the disabled or the Paralympic Sports Association. Amateur radio was his introduction to both. It brought people like Bob Steadward and Gerry Way and other officials of the wheelchair basketball championship games to the hospital to listen to the nation-wide hookup—"people who became very important" in Gary's life and who would introduce him to wheelchair sports, one of the greatest of all his contributions to the cause of the persons with disabilities.

12 | Cruel Blows

THEY HAD A GREAT ZEST FOR LIFE, the residents of Station 67, but for most of them the hold on life was tenuous, not due to any weakness of grip but rather to the fraying thread that seemed ready to snap at any time.

Some actually were, as the poet Keats once wrote, "half in love with easeful death." A former air force pilot, Don Neeland, was totally paralyzed, like Clayton, and completely dependent on the respirator. He had a devoted wife and twin sons about a year old; what on earth could he ever do to contribute to their well-being? On her first afternoon on shift, nursing aide Betty Fraser tried to lift Don up by his shoulders to remove his shirt. To her dismay, he "collapsed like a book" in her arms, such was the extreme wasting of his muscles. Don lived within himself and communicated with few people, but when Betty returned a few minutes later with tears drying on her cheeks, he too began to sob. Was it worth living like this? Don hung on until November 10, 1978, the day of his longed-for release from life.

Gary was in the midst of it. "Death was all around me, and I just couldn't grasp it," he said. One of the first losses was a totally unexpected death that laid teenaged Gary low in the pit of depression for days. Before getting a moderately severe form of polio, John Lagoyda was in his twenties and living in Raymond, Alberta, where he had gained a reputation as an excellent junior hockey player. His parents, of Czechoslovakian descent, often appeared on the ward with a tray of delicious cabbage, which Johnny shared with the rest of the boys in that room. One evening at 5:30 he suddenly collapsed and died on the spot. "In a flash he was gone," said Gary. Johnny Lagoyda escaped the long years of disability that lay before him; he died from a ruptured cerebral aneurysm and brain hemorrhage.

For Gary, there was a great sense of loss. He would lose more buddies, and the emotional trauma of their departing might blunt but never diminish. During such times the strong ties that bound together the "family" of polio survivors and their caregivers enabled them to stand together in their grief. Darlene Steljes, one of the first respiratory therapists at the University Hospital, lost her husband when he was only twenty-nine. "The people who helped me most to survive after his death were the patients on the polio ward," she said without hesitation. "They were there for me, my entire support system."

A few years down the road, another loss left Gary wondering if there was any justice at all in the universe. Sandy Burgess, who Gary greatly admired for his motivation and courage, was determined to pursue his education despite total paralysis from the neck down. Amazingly, he completed high school and then went on to university, acquiring his degree in law, doing all his typing and writing with his mouth. Later, while articling with his father's law firm in Camrose, he got engaged to a nurse. His old polio buddies were preparing to go to Camrose for a stag party for him. Sadly, two weeks before the marriage date, he got sick with fever, nausea and was just feeling unwell. Lacking any sensation below his neck, he felt no pain. Doctors struggled to make a diagnosis. In desperation, they finally took him to the operating room, but it was too late. His appendix had ruptured, and the spreading peritonitis took his life.

Arnie Stebner died in May, 1968. When the staff wheeled his bed out of the big ward to a side room, his friends followed anxiously with watchful eyes, fearful of the worst. For several days he had grown weaker and his breathing shallower. Everyone on the polio ward went to his funeral. The Stebner family, who had adopted the boys years before and endeared themselves to the whole ward, continued to pay for all the operating expenses of the red van.

Arnie's death had a remarkable effect on Gary. "He seemed to switch into high gear," his mother said. Before then, his efforts had been directed towards coping with his own disability and making the best of it. Henceforth, he would go to bat for others with disabilities. It seemed to be a "calling" that he could not ignore, even if the specifics were lacking. He would be an advocate and a crusader for the disabled.

13 | On the Road and in the Air

DURING HIS TEENAGE YEARS, Gary and his friends rarely missed an opportunity to leave the polio ward and get out and around, even if they were quite incapable of driving any kind of vehicle. After the age of twenty, Gary was travelling all over, always returning in due course to his hospital home on Station 67. Then, like an emerging butterfly, he was ready to try flying.

It started with a flight from Edmonton to Prince George, British Columbia, hardly a risky adventure for an able-bodied person but a bit of a challenge for a quadriplegic with impaired breathing. Dorothy and Rod McPherson had been transferred to Prince George, an important career move for Rod but one which made them both feel uneasy about leaving Gary. Far from neglecting him during his eleven years on the polio ward, they had proven remarkably faithful and supportive, visiting him often and bringing him home for short periods. With doubts filling their minds, they went ahead and invited Gary to come to Prince George for Christmas. When he arrived after the two-hour flight, they were surprised to find him calm and composed. A friend had helped get him aboard in Edmonton, and a stewardess had looked after him during the flight.

His motto thereafter became "Why not?" And when the opportunity to make a trip to Britain came up the following year, Gary seized it. His British grandmother had visited him in Edmonton in 1966. Before departing, she had invited him to "come on over." Though Gary looked upon it as a pretty casual invitation, Grandma Fleurie meant business, and the following year—when she was lucky enough to have won a large sum of money in a soccer pool—she repeated the invitation, offering to pay for his airfare and that of a companion, Doug Johnson, Bob's younger brother and a good friend.

Gary realized there would be perils and hazards. In those days, few people with disabilities travelled and wheelchair access to most buildings was limited or nonexistent. Suppose he ran into breathing difficulty en route? By this time he had learned to frog-breathe, but how would he fare during a lengthy airplane trip? He decided to take two chest respirators that could be hooked up to an electric motor. Then there was the problem of adapting the motor to the British power system, which used 220 volts. The British Polio Fellowship was contacted and they mailed an adaptor which arrived well before departure time. By this time Gary had learned the importance of foresight and careful preparation in whatever he did, and travelling by air, he wisely realized, needed special planning.

The thirty-four days in Britain were "red-letter days" for both Doug and Gary. Grandma Fleurie was a gracious hostess and took them to Portsmouth, Brighton and London, where they saw celebrated attractions such as the Tower of London and Buckingham Palace. They had been warned about the danger of trying to cross the busy London streets with a wheelchair and felt anxious about it. "We needn't have worried," said Gary. "The bobbies simply held up their hands and stopped the traffic for us." The British Polio Fellowship entertained them royally. After they arrived home on September 18, a reporter wrote, "Last to emerge [from the plane], a happy grin splitting his handsome features, was a young man borne in the arms of his husky young friend."[1]

The jaunt to England with Doug Johnson had a huge impact on Gary. It took away any fear of travelling and broadened his ever-widening horizons. He would use his experience on the airline many times to reassure and advise other disabled people preparing for a trip.

Dan Fortin was one of many attendants who escorted Gary on flights in years to come. Brushing his teeth, feeding him and putting him on the toilet were some of the tasks. "It was probably one of the best educational experiences I ever had," he said. Gary's wheelchair would be loaded with the regular baggage, and Dan would carry him up the stairs and into his seat. He was always the first to be boarded and the last to leave. On one occasion the ground staff provided a fork-lift with a platform to get Gary off the airplane.

Bob Steadward remembers one long trip when Gary, whose scoliosis made sitting uncomfortable, was clearly getting weary sitting in the upright position. Bob looked sideways and could see his companion having trouble breathing. He reached over and "bagged" him, pumping air into his lungs through a mouthpiece or a face mask. One time he took the long hose from his respirator and stuck it up next to the overhead air vent. Both methods seemed to work.

Once the pilot of an Air Canada plane departing from Toronto had to delay takeoff because of Gary McPherson. Gary had asked Gerry Way, at the time a colleague in the Paralympic Sports Association, to take him to the bathroom before the flight left. But there was a problem—it was a one-person toilet. Try as he might, Gerry could not close the door. So the stewardess held up a curtain in front of the open door during the whole operation, then took down the curtain and signalled to the pilot that he could take off.

On another occasion Gerry Way was travelling by train with Gary to a meeting in Toronto. The CNR had cooperated by providing their compartment with power for Gary's respirator. The two travellers kept their door open and chatted with other passengers walking through the corridor. One day, as Gerry was sitting in the compartment feeding Gary and himself, an air force nursing sister passed by, stopped and came inside. She asked a few questions, then put her arm around Gary and asked, "Do you mind if I feed you?" Of course, neither one of them could object, and they gained a new friend.

He had no trouble meeting strangers. Karen O'Neill of Ottawa worked with Gary in wheelchair sports when she was director-general of the Canadian Wheelchair Sports Association (CWSA). Once the two of them were in the lobby of the Westin hotel when Karen had to leave for another appointment. She apologized, knowing that Gary was on his own and didn't know anyone around. "That's okay," he said. "I'll make some new friends."

Travelling gave him many new friends and bountiful experiences, some good and some otherwise. His escorts invariably said that they were all good learning experiences and that Gary nearly always found something positive, encouraging and thought-provoking.

·　·　·　·　·

IT WAS THE MIDDLE OF WINTER, and everyone on the polio ward was tired of looking out at ice and snow. Many of those with respiratory polio declined invitations to go out, fearing exposure to wintry winds and frost-laden air. All were feeling cooped up and housebound.

Ron Fortin remembers how it all started. He had just lifted Gary from his wheelchair and plunked him onto the toilet. He then sat himself back in the wheelchair and pondered.

"You know, Gary, we should do something. We should pick up this whole ward and go to Hawaii or some place."

"Really?" said Gary.

He sat there for a while, eyebrows raised and lips pursed quizzically. Go to Hawaii? Lovely idea, but—people with disabilities didn't travel much in those days, and for a group of them to travel together—well, that would be next to impossible. Maybe to Calgary or even Vancouver, but not to Hawaii for a flight of seven to eight hours with a bunch of paralyzed people dependent on respirators for their breathing.

Many of them—staff and patients—had seen others' photographs of palm trees and beautiful sandy beaches and dreamed about going to those idyllic islands themselves. But could that dream ever come true? Hardly likely.

But the idea just wouldn't go away. Gary couldn't dismiss it outright—he had already flown to England with his friend Doug Johnson and travelled to Heidelberg, Germany, in 1972 for the Twenty-first International Stoke Mandeville Games (the 1972 Paralympic Games), in addition to other trips for wheelchair sports. Each trip had required careful planning and preparation. The logistics of a group trip to Hawaii would be daunting. Daunting, but maybe just possible. As the idea began to fly around the polio ward like their budgie of a previous year, more and more people nodded their heads in agreement. Looking back, Gary said, "I guess naïvety is sometimes a good thing. We sure didn't realize what a major project it would prove to be."

Every time they made enquiries, the more plausible it became. They started by approaching hospital administration, who seemed startled but not totally opposed to the request. They would sanction the trip, provided they could be assured all the minute details had been scrupulously worked out. In retrospect, Gary believes they thought it would never take place.

The planners figured that the biggest mountain to climb would be transportation. But they were lucky enough to have a contact right on the ward, in fact, one of the "boys." A woman named Doreen Rouse, an almost-weekly visitor to Clayton for several years, was the executive assistant to Max Ward of Wardair. She knew many of the polio survivors and understood what they would need in terms of assisted respiration during the flight. Through Doreen, a meeting was held with Wardair officials, who gave tentative approval to the trip.

Fund-raising would be a major challenge. To minimize the burden for those with limited resources, each of the would-be travellers was asked to raise only four hundred dollars. Needing to raise an additional eighteen thousand dollars, the committee approached some of Gary's connections in the Jaycees, locals of the hospital unions, Rotary Club members and Edmonton's Civic Welfare Chest Fund. They made it clear they were not seeking money for charity but rather for a project that would brighten the lives of seriously disabled, hospital-bound polio survivors. Moved by the objectives and the uniqueness of the project, donors gave generously; convinced of its merits, they wanted to be part of it.

Next came the nitty-gritty details. Gary wanted—insofar as it was possible—to make the journey risk-free for the thirteen respiratory-assisted polio patients, men and women, wanting to go. To provide the necessary support, he recruited eighteen staff and escorts to accompany them, making a total of thirty-one travellers, including John Reader, a medical technician from the Aberhart, Darlene Steljes, a respiratory therapist, and Jim Archibald, a resident in pulmonary medicine. A number of the patients could get by without their respirators for only two to three hours, a potentially serious problem for a long flight. Wardair agreed not only to make their oxygen supply available but also to provide power outlets for the respirators. Darlene devised a Y-shaped connection so that two people could use one respirator.

Arrangements at the Hawaii end demanded even more forethought. They would need accommodation at a suitable hotel with wheelchair access. A friend in one of the Edmonton Kiwanis Clubs contacted a club member in Honolulu who, in turn, approached the Sheraton hotel. The management agreed to accommodate the respiratory polio patients and their escorts for two weeks at much reduced rates. Then it was a question of arranging appropriate transportation in Hawaii, a supply of oxygen, batteries for the respirators (when away from the hotel room) and preparations for potential medical requirements.

It looked like a reconnaissance flight would be necessary. Ron Fortin and Gary volunteered to go—without much persuasion—and Wardair provided free airline tickets. The Honolulu Kiwanis Club arranged for free accommodation for them at the Sheraton Waikiki. Arriving in January, Ron and Gary took several days to arrange for ground transportation, batteries and an oxygen supply from a medical supply house. They finalized arrangements with the Sheraton for thirty-one guests for a two-week period. They even approached the Queen's Medical Center, to be sure of a backup in case of a medical emergency. It just so happened that the local Wardair representative was Cheryl Regan, who had been a stewardess onboard the flight that took Gary and his friend Doug Johnson to England in 1967. Gary, never one to forget an attractive young lady, recognized her right away. Cheryl helped them greatly with their plans before they returned to Edmonton. Then followed a series of orientation sessions, focusing mainly on safety.

Excitement was running high on the morning of March 2 when the group of thirty-one took off from wintry Edmonton. Supplies of power and oxygen were abundant throughout the long journey. Everyone breathed more or less normally, except for some hyperventilation when the white sands and blue waters of the Hawaiian Islands hove into view.

If the planning and arranging had weighed heavily at times, the rewards in terms of the pleasure and happiness of a Hawaiian holiday made it all worthwhile. For many of the patients it was undoubtedly a dream come true; for staff (still on salary, but not entirely on duty), it was a grand holiday. They toured around and visited beauty spots and historical sights, lazed on the beach or had fun together in the living room of Gary's suite at the hotel. After a couple of days, all the patients seemed to improve dramatically. "It was like they got an infusion of life," Darlene said. "They seemed to forget their anxieties and worries, the product of the dehumanizing influence of the hospital." And the thorough precautionary measures paid off: no one got sick except for Henri Baril, who developed a temporary problem with blockage of his eustachian tube. "Everything went off without a hitch," Gary said, "like a NASA space flight."

The unusual group of visitors had not anticipated the splash they would make on the local scene. When Honolulu newspapers learned of the unique adventure, they ran a column in two issues.[2] The Hawaii State Legislature even recognized and honored the organizers of "Project Hawaii" during a session.[3]

Soon after the group returned to Edmonton, Max Ward and Gary McPherson were honoured with a certificate of merit from the Alberta Medical Association.[4] Gary calls it one of the biggest projects he was ever involved in. Each of the thirty-one travellers regarded it as "a feather in his cap." Dr. Bob Fraser, one of first physicians to care for Gary, shook his head incredulously, calling the whole Hawaii trip "a phenomenal piece of activity."

The success of the project was in itself sufficient reward for Gary, who had provided most of the drive and intricate planning. But far more meaningful was the knowledge that it had given such pleasure to people he had lived with for so many years, people he called "my extended family." In particular, Don Neeland hadn't been on a holiday with his wife since he got polio in 1955. A taciturn fellow who struggled to cope with his serious disability, he seemed on better terms with life after the Hawaii trip.

14 | The Butterfly Emerges from Its Chrysalis

We believe that faith in God gives purpose and meaning to human life; the brotherhood of man transcends the sovereignty of nations; economic justice can best be won by free men through free enterprise; government should be of laws rather than of men; earth's greatest treasure lives in human personality; service to humanity is the best work of life.

—CREED OF THE JUNIOR CHAMBER OF COMMERCE

IT ALL STARTED with an ad in the *Edmonton Journal* and the phone call that followed.

"This is Gary McPherson speaking. I read about the Patterson sales seminar and would like to know more. I understand it's sponsored by the Edmonton Jaycees."

"Hi, Gary. This is George de Rappard from the Jaycees. If you're interested, I could meet you at the lobby of the Jubilee Auditorium before it begins."

"Fine," said Gary, "but I'll need a ride."

George arranged a ride and met Gary as planned. He was taken aback to see a young fellow with limbs like matchsticks sitting in a wheelchair, totally paralyzed except for slight movement in his left hand and leg. But he seemed bright enough and keen on learning more about the Jaycees. George then wheeled him into the auditorium for the start of the presentation. Gary was not so much interested in salesmanship as he was in the Jaycees themselves. He had learned about the personal development courses and other activities offered by the Junior Chamber of Commerce. The newspaper ad displayed photos and testimonials that had piqued his interest; something inside him said, "Go!" He was twenty-one and felt like a rudderless ship, the direction of his life still vague and nebulous. The Patterson seminar provided the introduction he needed to the activities of the Jaycees. To this day he remembers what one speaker said about quality: "If your family is important to you, don't ride on bad tires. People or things that are important to you deserve the best."

George de Rappard, then president of the Jaycees, took a liking to Gary, told him about the activities of the Jaycees and welcomed him to become a member. To get him involved, he invited Gary to join the committee on public relations, chaired by Al Menard. George introduced him to other members who offered to give Gary a ride to meetings any time. Soon Gary found himself attending meetings regularly and even arranged for the odd meeting to be held at the hospital.

He took every personal development and growth course that the Jaycees offered, which included effective speaking, leadership training, parliamentary procedure and budgeting. When the time came to make a speech in front of his colleagues, he felt considerable disquietude. "I just knew I would make a fool out of myself." Of course, he couldn't make notes beforehand and had to rely on a helper to jot down his ideas.

Further, when they were selecting topics for the talks, Gary began to realize what he called the shallowness of his knowledge. His colleagues were careful to critique him in a firm but gentle way, but he still realized the flimsiness of content in his talks. Sometimes he had to speak "off the cuff" and that forced him to think quickly. He persisted, and a year later he was teaching the effective speaking course to student nurses at the Royal Alexandra Hospital.

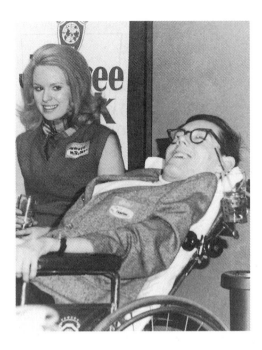

Gary with "Miss Edmonton," Heather McRoberts during Jaycee Week in 1969.

For three years he was completely involved. "He embraced the organization, which in turn embraced him," George de Rappard said. Gary attended a couple of conventions, entered speaking competitions, took all the theory courses offered and ended up chairing three commissions: membership, public relations and leadership training. He studied the basics of parliamentary procedure but claims he never mastered *Robert's Rules of Order.*

The Jaycees' philosophy included the belief that members learn by active participation. As a commission member, Gary was free to originate a community project, do the research and the organizing, then present it to the board of directors. If the board approved, the project could be implemented. There was plenty of room for initiative, but of course he would be held accountable. Al Menard remembers Gary's committee work. "When Gary was on a committee, we could tell him what needed to be done and then we could forget it. It would be done."

Bob and Doug Johnson joined the Jaycees for a while, as did Beaver—all at Gary's instigation, but none became so deeply immersed. People with disabilities were readily accepted, even though the inaccessibility of the organization's dinner meetings meant having to lug wheelchairs up and down a flight of twenty-six steps. For the first year or so, Gary deliberately ate his supper before going out, in order to save money and to avoid the need for someone to feed him. Later, when many members were offering to feed him, he gave in. But they didn't offer him any other privileges, and as he gained their respect, they treated him as they would anyone else.

There came a time, however, when being treated as an equal was overwhelming and just a trifle anxiety-producing. One of the fellows volunteered to take Gary home in his little Triumph TR sports car. He plunked Gary into the passenger seat, then drove off, steering with one hand and with the other clutching the wheelchair, which was slithering around precariously on the back of the car. As they rounded one corner, the wheelchair almost flew away. Happily, Gary got back to the hospital intact—slightly thankful to his devil-may-care driver and very thankful to have avoided a mishap.

Did the Jaycees groom people for politics or somehow attract people of any political inclination? George de Rappard became chief deputy minister under Premier Peter Lougheed and worked out of his office. Another member, Cec Purves, was mayor of Edmonton from 1977 to 1983. Gary took out a membership in the Conservative party soon after joining the Jaycees but never activated it until he had left.

The Jaycees provided valuable training ground for Gary and showed him that he could make a worthy contribution to the community outside of the University Hospital. He became convinced he could "compete in the real world." And compete he did, running for office in the Jaycees' annual election (conducted much like a political election) and winning a place on the board of directors, where he was responsible for the leadership development committee. Then in 1971 he was elected to the executive as secretary-treasurer.

The next year the question was raised: How about running for president? He, and others, believed he could have handled the job, but he declined, fearing that the stresses on his weakened and frail body would simply be too much.

Beaver recalls his time with the Jaycees as happy, learning times with a great bunch of fellows. Gary is convinced that the three and a half years with the Jaycees was "pivotal to my career." Their programs and meetings were people-oriented and more to his liking than working at computers. He gained confidence, a new network of friends, contacts with the community, self-esteem and a facility in public speaking. The latter was a great accomplishment—a sterling victory that saw him overcome the challenges of a paralyzed diaphragm and an inability to make notes. In fact, he placed second to the man who went on to win the national competition in public speaking. Almost as valuable was the skill he acquired in chairing a meeting and following an agenda. George de Rappard had no doubt that "the Jaycees turned his life around. They helped remove 'the hedges and barriers of hospital existence,' developed in him a positive attitude and fortified his feeling of self-worth."

· · · · ·

GARY HAD BECOME A TOKEN MEMBER of the Conservative party, but a deep suspicion of the political process, including the bickering, haggling and prejudice, kept politics at the periphery of his interests. His long years of dependency in hospital had taught him the importance of tolerance and respect—attitudes as rare as comets in political circles.

But soon after leaving the Jaycees in 1971, his lukewarm interest began to heat up. The Progressive Conservatives, after long years of sitting in the provincial legislature in opposition, started to engender interest and support among the electorate. At that stage the PCs held only a half-dozen seats, three of the members being Peter Lougheed, Don Getty and Lou Hyndman. What particularly impressed Gary, an undying sports fan, was that two of the leading lights, Lougheed and Getty, had played football. A few short years before, Getty had been quarterback for the Edmonton Eskimos. What better reasons to support a political party?

After Premier Harry Strom called an election, Gary phoned the PC headquarters and learned that Getty was running for re-election in his area. He had met him briefly at the racetrack years before and knew little about the man, but he thought the Conservatives were on the move and he wanted to be part of the movement. Getty's campaign headquarters was located in a trailer on 114 Street, south of University Avenue; if Gary wanted to volunteer, that's where he would have to go. Not a very impressive place, but fortunately fairly close to the University Hospital.

Gary phoned his young brother, Roddy, who was only ten at the time and on summer holidays, and recruited him to push his wheelchair down to the campaign office. This routine prevailed every day until school started. Among other jobs, Roddy answered the phone, saying, "Good morning, this is Don Getty's headquarters" in as deep a voice as he could muster. For his efforts, he was paid ten cents an hour by his mother.

Gary arrived as a volunteer, new at the job but with some experience arising from his involvement in the Jaycees' elections. With Roddy as his helper, he was ready and willing to do whatever was needed, within the realm of his capabilities. After a few days, "they designated me as office manager." Gary claims that he rated that job only because he was always in the office, whereas others came and went. Access to and from the trailer by wheelchair was difficult until someone built a ramp.

Working with the many volunteers, he quickly got his finger on the pulse for the eight weeks of intense campaign activities. Don Getty dropped into the office every day, but he spent most of his time else-where, making speeches and knocking on doors.

The PCs won the election in a landslide, unseating the long-standing Social Credit government. Lougheed, leader of the party, became premier, and Getty, the minister of energy. Gary's mentor in the Jaycees, George de Rappard, was appointed by Premier Lougheed first as executive-director of the Progressive Conservative Association of Alberta and then as chief deputy minister. Percy Wickman, a wheelchair-using MLA on the other side of the house, marvelled that a person so seriously handicapped as Gary could handle the job of office manager for Getty's campaign. "The key to an effective political campaign is good office coordination," he said. "Gary deserves a lot of credit for that."

After weeks of close association between the candidate and his office manager, a mutual respect and admiration had developed, progressing to an enduring friendship. Don Getty described Gary's efforts as "a real inspiration to all the people working to get me elected." When he later visited Gary at the Aberhart, he was surprised to find his room a hive of activity. He realized how deeply involved Gary had becomes in the community outside the hospital.

In later years Don Getty would find himself marching happily along with advocacy groups working for persons with disability. But Gary was not his first contact with a person confined to a wheelchair because of respiratory polio. Don Getty hunted ducks with Ray Allison, a fellow employee with Imperial Oil in the early 1950s. Ray's wife Elaine got polio during the epidemic of 1953, spent four years in hospital and then went home, relying on a rocking bed and pneumobelt (an inflatable belt with alternating pressure) to help with her breathing. Ray kept his wife at home for many years, hiring a housekeeper on a regular basis and lifting her to and from her wheelchair himself. Her breathing improved, and with her right hand she did petit-point pictures and operated a computer keyboard.

During those difficult years, Ray Allison struggled to keep his head above water. Until 1973, he received only seventy-five dollars a month from the Alberta government. With the encouragement of his friend Don Getty, then minister of energy, he and Gary McPherson approached Bill Rawson, a deputy minister in the Department of Social Services, asking for support for home care. Gary cited the case of Henri and Liz Baril, whose marriage might have been happier and Henri's life prolonged had they been provided with help in the home. Ray even threatened to seek readmission to hospital for Elaine if home support was not forth-coming.

Soon afterwards the "Polio Program" legislation was passed to assist in the home care of respiratory polio survivors and to provide grants to build wheelchair ramps and railings. Initially Ray received an allowance of $500 a month, a figure that was later increased to $750. Connie Clarke, afflicted with disability comparable to Gary's, received $1,200 because she needed full-time help. The government department had to be convinced first that home care was really more cost-effective than institutional care.

Don Getty has long since left politics, with few regrets. During the latter months of his term as premier, he was the butt of much scathing criticism and fault-finding. Gary maintains that much of it was unde-served and that, if anything, he should have been more hard-nosed and ruthless. He calls Don "a sincere, caring sort of person who would go to the wall for you." To this day they remain friends.

15 | The Hospital

Home Base for Sports for the Disabled

FOR THE FIRST FEW YEARS, no one on polio wards 32 and 67 doubted that Gary should remain a patient at the University Hospital. Even so, it was a tough decision—at times he longed to go home, and his parents were still hopeful that they would be able to look after him.

But as time passed, it became abundantly clear that the decision to stay was the right one. Although Gary had learned frog-breathing, he still used a ventilator, especially at night. Nothing could replace the presence of trained staff on hand and properly functioning devices for assisted breathing.

Eric Boyd, a wheelchair athlete and later Gary's associate on the Premier's Council on the Status of Persons with Disabilities, had no hesitation in describing respirator-dependency as "the epitome of insecurity." In Vancouver during the 1973 Canadian Wheelchair Games, Gary was dragged into the clutches of that terrible insecurity in the middle of the night. He was trying to sleep in the dormitory room next to his brother Scott when his respirator failed. By the time Scott roused, Gary was desperate. But from previous contact over amateur radio, he knew there was a polio unit in Vancouver, and he got Scott to phone. They quickly despatched a taxi with a replacement respirator to the university dormitory. It worked reasonably well, but Gary got little sleep.

The least incapacitated of the boys, Beaver was the first to move out of hospital. He had started working part-time in 1974, being driven between the hospital and his job. In 1980, when his employer, Canadian Utilities, hired him full-time for his data processing skills, he felt confident enough to leave hospital for good. Although Beaver received no financial help except for token support from the Canadian Legion's Polio Foundation, he acquired the financial security that his buddy lacked; the income from Gary's work with wheelchair sports was little more than a pittance.

Not everyone admired Gary for his unwillingness to step out from the safe and sheltered existence of hospital life. Other disabled people had left the institutional life, quietly got an education and become self-supporting, working in a competitive society. "He's no hero," they said, resenting his living in the comfortable hospital environment for years on end at taxpayers' expense and getting far more public acclaim than they thought he deserved.

But such voices were few. In the light of all his contributions, Gary could hardly be considered a parasite. Not only was he aware of the life-threatening risks, he had witnessed the heartaches and tragedies that befell similar patients who had left hospital without essential support. Henri Baril, one of the remaining "boys" still living, married a beautiful and warm-hearted student nurse, Liz, in 1972. Henri's disability was even more severe than Gary's, but he had learned frog-breathing and developed much skill as a mouth-painter. Liz and Henri seemed like an ideal couple, but their marriage was anything but happy. Try as she might, Liz could simply not cope: the stresses and strains of day-after-day demands as a hospital nurse, housewife and caregiver to a pleasant but seriously disabled husband wore her down. She and Henri would openly fight and argue in Gary's presence. "It just wasn't like them at all," said Gary. They had a couple of children, much loved by their parents, but the stresses just grew. They remained together, living under duress, until Henri got pneumonia and had to return to hospital, this time to the Aberhart. There he died, the third member of the original boys to succumb.

By 1973, the polio ward—patients and staff—had moved from Station 67 in the University Hospital to the Aberhart Hospital, a sort of auxiliary to the university and connected to it, temporarily, by an underground tunnel. Station 67 was needed for more acute medical care beds, and one of the rooms formerly used for polio patients was being converted into an intensive care unit.

Some of the long-term patients were glad to make the move; some were not. It was like moving from a big city with lots of ongoing activity to a small, sleepy town. What's more, nearly all the staff knew or recognized the old-timers, and many had become friends.

Built as a tuberculosis sanatorium, the Aberhart found patient numbers shrinking; effective medication controlled the once-dangerous disease, allowing many patients to go home. Now only the fourth floor was set aside for TB patients. A rehab ward (formerly Station 66 of the University Hospital) was established on the third floor, while long-term polio patients and those with other respiratory ailments, like emphysema and asthma, got the first floor.

In some respects it was a good move for the patients. They could look out the window and see green grass and flowers blossoming at eye level. There was more privacy and the opportunity to develop a homelike atmosphere. If they had to be moved, the veteran polio patients were ready to use the occasion to lay down demands for relaxation of hospital rules. For the most part they got their way, including such privileges as unlimited visiting hours and overnight guests.

No longer were ten fellows confined in close proximity in one large room; most of the rooms had four beds, and in the case of Clayton May and Bob Johnson, only two. Beaver and Gary were together in one room, two old buddies who got along well but saw each other rarely, "like ships passing in the night." Beaver worked part-time at Canadian Utilities, and Gary was often away on some business to do with wheelchair sports. Life was quieter and better organized, but they all missed the fellowship of the "family meals" on Station 67 when all food trays were wheeled in on

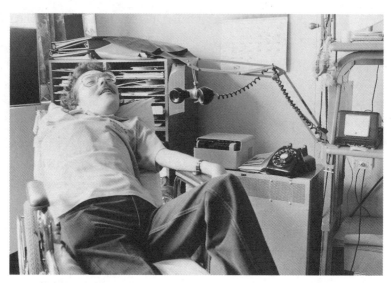

Gary's office in the Aberhart Hospital served as his base of operations in his role as executive-director of the Canadian Wheelchair Sports Association (CWSA).

a stretcher. The chit-chat, laughter and good fellowship of the communal meal was lost.

Set apart from the others, Beaver and Gary went on to develop their own interests and lifestyles. The new hospital room became for Gary more than a home; it grew into an office. He had a fair-sized L-shaped desk, filing cabinets and a special phone that he could answer by hitting a switch with his knee. His mother came in every day and helped with secretarial work.

There were staff on hand, but otherwise the hospital environment was hardly evident. No longer considering himself a patient, Gary drew up his own schedule and aimed to control his own activities, which under-standably, "created resistance and friction." But being almost totally dependent on others, he could not bulldoze his way. He had long since learned the importance of respecting people; now he could carry that lesson further and learn to assess the personalities of people and how they responded. And in time he was able to say, "The more interaction we had with the administration, the more two-way respect we had."

Eric Boyd described the Aberhart as a prison without bars for Gary, but also a place of great security where all his needs were met. According to Eric, what people with disabilities generally want from society is "the support to allow us to be independent and to live with dignity in the community." Gary had that in the Aberhart. He used it as a base for his many activities but probably would have moved out before he did, had he been able to get the necessary home care and support. He was determined not to go until that was in place.

Soon after moving to the Aberhart, Gary became executive-director of the Canadian Wheelchair Sports Association (CWSA). A flood of documents and papers soon covered the entire surface of his desk. He could get up in the morning and go to work, sometimes for a couple of hours, sometimes for the entire day.

Percy Wickman, a paraplegic and former MLA in the Alberta government, was once a long-term patient in an institution. He said, "The institution can zap your brains and suck out all your initiative." Some patients withdraw into an inert submissive state; others just give up, wither away and die. Fortunately, there are exceptions. Lea Sanderson, a volunteer who met Gary soon after the move to the Aberhart, said, "He is a perfect example of how independent a severely disabled person can be, in spite of being trapped in a hospital for so long."

Gary looks back with appreciation for those long years in hospital, viewing that time as "a rich, diverse experience" and holding most of the staff, patients and volunteers in high regard. He learned a lot—from a position of weakness—about human dynamics and interaction, negotiating differences and dealing with people in authority. It all helped towards his growth and development. And he is thankful to the people of Alberta who, through government social programs, enabled him to live and work in a hospital institution.

As Ron Fortin, orderly on the Aberhart for five years, put it: "He may have been a prisoner, but he flew with the eagles."

· · · · ·

SINCE CHILDHOOD Gary had had a passion for sport of all kinds, and after the death of his close buddy Arnie in 1968, he resolved to take up the cause of the disabled. But he had no inkling then that these two consuming interests might roll into one: sporting activities for persons with disability. And it might never have happened, had Gary and his pals not provided the essential radio communications for the 1968 Wheelchair Games in Edmonton, a helping hand that resulted in a certificate of merit for the amateur radio operators.

The local Paralympic Sports Association (PSA), which included a wheelchair athlete called Stu Warrior, remembered that good piece of work. A double above-knee amputee, Stu had been a member of the Jaycees and as such had some idea of what Gary could and could not do. He approached him some time in 1971, soon after Gary had left the Jaycees.

"How about running for president of the PSA?" he asked.

"But I know very little about your organization," Gary replied.

"That's okay. I've seen you at work. If you'll run, I'd be willing to be your campaign manager."

Gary consented. The election was scheduled for the upcoming annual meeting, but he contracted pneumonia, was confined to his bed for three weeks and couldn't attend. Stu Warrior must have done a good job of campaigning—Gary won easily against his opponent.

After recovering from pneumonia, he began his two-year term, set to work and was delighted with what he found. The first PSA president, Gerry Way, had provided excellent leadership and proved a great help to his successor. Gary found the association to have "a vibrant membership," all of whom were volunteers. His old friend Bob Steadward served as athletic director. Gary's main work was in administration: recruiting members, working on public relations, promoting basketball programs, building up profile and raising funds.

Edmonton's PSA was one of the leading groups for disabled sports in the country at that time. Working primarily in wheelchair sports, it focused mainly on programs for people with spinal injuries and polio, but also included those with cerebral palsy and amputees. Gary considers his succession to the presidency of PSA as one of a handful of "defining moments" in his life.

After his election, he made a special request for a secretary. So Dorothy, the mother with whom he had always had a warm relationship, was appointed to the job. Dorothy accepted, wanting to be supportive of Gary, even though she was busy enough with a full-time job and raising her children. They developed into an efficient and harmonious mother-son team. When Gary moved on, Dorothy "became involved on my own behalf" with PSA and served for more than twenty years as a volunteer.

Before 1966, there was no organized approach to sport or recreation for disabled people in Edmonton. Then a meeting was called of volunteer groups like the Legion, the Scouts and the Canadian Paraplegic Association. Gerry Way attended as a delegate from the Scouts association and subsequently became a member of a steering committee. Six months later he left the Scouts to work full-time as a volunteer in the newly formed Paralympic Sports Association, designed to provide both sporting activities and recreation for people using wheelchairs. Their major endeavour was the 1968 Edmonton wheelchair games, where Gerry Way had the big job of arranging transportation. The games were highly successful, a feather in the cap of the young PSA organization.

It had taken one man to provide the impetus and drive to mobilize sports for the disabled at the national level. Dr. Bob Jackson, later to become team doctor for the Toronto Argonauts, attended the Paralympic Games in Japan in 1964; he saw some great paraplegic athletes, none of whom were Canadian. He returned to Canada, determined to make changes. He knew there were what he called "isolated pockets" for disabled athletes: organizations in Montreal, Toronto, Winnipeg and Edmonton, all functioning independently. He was determined to do his best to bring them all together.

Under Bob Jackson's leadership, the first meeting of Canadian Wheelchair Sports Association (CWSA) was held at the Pan-American

Games in Winnipeg in 1967. Thereafter the organization grew in dimension, strength and cohesiveness, with basketball being the most popular of about twelve sports, including track and field, archery, shooting and swimming. Dr. Jackson served as president of CWSA until his retirement in 1973.

As president of Edmonton's PSA group, Gary found himself being drawn more and more into sports for the disabled. He and Athletic Director Bob Steadward were aiming high: they hoped and planned to hold the 1976 "Olympics for the Disabled" (as they were called) in Edmonton. They had the needed leadership and fine facilities at the University of Alberta. To learn all they could, in 1972 they travelled, along with Gerry Way, to Heidelberg, Germany, where the International Stoke Mandeville Games were being held. Gary's brother Scott travelled with him and served as his attendant for the two weeks they were away.

While they failed in their attempt—the 1976 Paralympics went to Toronto, not Edmonton—they didn't feel discouraged. "It was a growth experience," said Gary. "We learned a lot by just being there, seeing how things were done, and meeting people from other countries involved in wheelchair sports."

When the pioneering Dr. Jackson retired as president of the CWSA, he was succeeded by Dr. Maury Van Vliet, director of physical education at the University of Alberta. Gerry Way, who had been working as executive-director entirely as a volunteer, decided to move on. So in 1974 the board of directors approached Gary McPherson to take over as executive-director of the national organization. It was an awesome undertaking for a man unable to write a single word, but here again, faithful Dorothy offered to help.

Operating from an "office" at the Aberhart Hospital, Gary's job entailed keeping in touch with all provincial branches, maintaining liaison with government departments and applying for grants. It offered no remuneration but provided expenses. The hospital room that he shared with Beaver became virtually the centre for wheelchair sports. Gary found himself making trips to Ottawa to lobby on behalf of wheelchair sports, to convince the authorities that the CWSA was a bona fide sporting organization. He made it clear that his goal was to raise the level of performance of Canada's wheelchair athletes so they could be more effective in international competitions.

After two and a half years on the job, federal government funding was secured to provide an executive-director's salary. But raising the status of CWSA meant relocating the office to Ottawa, a move that Gary was unwilling to make.

So in 1978, he reluctantly said farewell—temporarily—to the national organization. For the previous seven years he had "lived, eaten and breathed wheelchair sport." He devoted four years of that period to leading a national organization without much more than his personal passion and the help of others across Canada who believed in wheelchair sport. As Darryl Rock, author of *Making a Difference: Profiles in Abilities,* wrote, "What he lacked in resources he more than made up for in creativity, ingenuity and by calling on his vast network of colleagues from coast to coast."[1]

Gary may have left the helm of the CWSA ship in 1978, but he showed himself willing to be a part of the national organization by serving as volunteer treasurer for a couple of years thereafter, followed in 1984 by an eight-year stretch as president. He was involved in the 1978 Commonwealth Games and the 1983 World University Games, both held in Edmonton.

Peter Eriksson, a member of Sweden's national speed-skating team in the 1970s, later went on to coach disabled athletes, men and women he considered "the real elite" because of the disability they refuse to give in to. He greatly admired Gary's long record of battling for a better chance for these heroic people. Thus far, Gary had devoted his best efforts, using his considerable administrative skills, towards "developing opportunities for athletes with disabilities."

But he would do more. A couple of years later he received an invitation that would offer him dramatic and fulfilling involvement with wheelchair basketball that he never would have imagined.

16 | Wheelchair Basketball and the Great Alberta Northern Lights

Certainly it has been shown in much research that, while sport has value in anyone's life, it is even more important in the life of a person with a disability. This is because of sport's rehabilitative influence, and the fact that it is a means to integrate the person into society.

—DR. BOB STEADWARD

President, International Paralympic Committee[1]

FOR FOUR YEARS, until he retired in 1978, Executive-secretary Gary McPherson's "office" at the Aberhart Hospital had been the heartbeat of the Canadian Wheelchair Sport Association (CWSA). During those busy years his daily tasks included accounting, administration, correspondence, fund-raising, board meetings, arranging travel for athletes and volunteers, coordinating programs and competitions. The job gobbled up his hours, but he loved it. But when the decision was made to relocate the CWSA "headquarters" to the National Sport and Recreation Centre in Ottawa, Gary gave up the job, not wanting to move from Edmonton.

Then he had to make another decision. Totally committed to working for the cause of society's disabled, he wondered what kind of efforts would

91

make the greatest impact. Though convinced of the value of sports of all kinds, he wondered about using political means and connections. Very, very few people with disabilities were involved in the political process, and even fewer in a proactive sense. Mostly they were agitating for assistance or handouts or services from governments or various agencies; efforts towards integration of the disabled into the mainstream of society were minimal. Gary gave serious consideration to joining the small coterie of activists but finally decided against it. "Political action is always so negative and fraught with complaining people," he said.

Not so with sport. He believed wheelchair sport to be a positive, constructive activity that probably created beneficial social change more effectively than social agitation. His ideas would, in due course, change, but at that point, "that is where I felt useful to myself and others."

The time had come for more involvement, more contact with the athletes whose welfare had become so important to him. Wheelchair basketball would provide that outlet. He had seen enough of that exciting sport to see the incredible benefits it conferred on players and volunteers, in fact, on everyone involved in any way. He stood at the threshold of an opportunity to be the chief architect in building a team of international stature.

It all began in 1972 when Reg McClellan, a young fellow working in pipeline construction near Red Deer, was hit in the back by heavy equipment, leaving him with a severe spinal injury and permanent paralysis. During his recovery he wandered down from Station 66, the rehab ward in the University Hospital, to the polio ward, where he met Clayton, Arnie, Beaver and Gary. "They were involved in all kinds of ventures," he remembers. After eight weeks Reg left hospital in a wheelchair, but not before getting fired up about wheelchair sports. "Gary was the one who introduced me to it," he said. Before his injury, Reg had played hockey for hours on end, but sporting activities for anyone using a wheelchair was to him an entirely new idea.

Over the next couple of years, Reg and Gary spent a lot of time planning and scheming, discussing ways to enhance opportunities for disabled people in the Edmonton area. At that time many people considered that the disabled athlete should be versatile, capable of taking part in several sporting events. Reg, however, favoured specialization, which would allow an athlete the chance to really excel. He found wheelchair basketball every bit as challenging and rewarding as hockey, and he soon began playing competitively. Setting high goals for himself, he travelled to Vancouver on some weekends to play for that city's team in a league known as the NWBA (North American Wheelchair Basketball Association).

But all the while he wondered what Edmonton might do to build a team. Was it just a dream to have a team good enough to participate in the NWBA? No league existed in Canada. The Paralympic Sports Association (PSA) had money in the bank, but the emphasis then was more on rehabilitation of the disabled than on sporting activities. Reg took out a mortgage on his house and got into a fund-raising campaign with a friend, Boots Cooper. They raised the money needed to launch a team and then began to recruit players.

In 1978, Reg and his entourage invited Gary to come onboard as general manager of the embryo team. Their reasons? "Gary had a similar vision. We both thought the sky was the limit. I knew him to be a meticulous organizer with the ability to enlist whatever help and support was needed." Their goal was to develop the best team in Canada. Apart from a mixed bag of athletes with varying degrees of skill and disability, they didn't have much going for them. They had no organization, no infrastructure, no support mechanisms and few volunteers. It would be a major venture into the almost-unknown.

Reclining in the wheelchair in his "office" at the Aberhart Hospital, Gary envisaged the practicalities of his job description. It would first involve establishing the organization as a nonprofit society and then recruiting a board of directors. He would have to build on Reg's work in fund-raising—contacting the business community and other sources. The recruitment of staff, athletes, referees and playing facilities would also be part of it.

Gary began by defining a mission statement, in simple terms showing the worthiness of the enterprise. The fund-raising was far from being a one-man campaign; the athletes played an active role. Ron Minor, one of the better-known disabled players, appeared at several public speaking events, making contact with private and corporate donors.

Premier Don Getty, a noteworthy basketball and football player of previous years, had visited Gary at the Aberhart Hospital several times and gotten to know many of the patients and nurses. He was only too happy to help raise money for the new team, having watched wheelchair basketball and calling it "an astonishing game." Later, he joined the board of directors, serving as honorary chairman.

It would be called the Alberta Northern Lights Wheelchair Basketball Team, a name suggested by Bob Steadward during a Saturday morning coffee session with some PSA members. Although most of the players came from northern Alberta, it would, in effect, be a provincial team.

To start with, they were for the most part "a ragtag bunch of guys," Gary said, many of them on welfare or worker's compensation. Most players were local, with a couple from Saskatchewan. They played whenever they could find an opposing team. Later a loosely held league existed with teams from Spokane and Vancouver. But the Lights, as they were known, had to do all the travelling; they rated little respect from other teams and were unsuccessful in getting them to come to Edmonton.

Early on, Gary set about building a board of directors. Blessed with a long list of contacts, he aimed for competent people and some high-profile community members. Rollie Miles of Edmonton Eskimos football fame was one of the first directors. Charlie Gardner, a young lawyer, got a phone call from Gary, but he wasn't overly enthusiastic about serving on the board. After a few more calls, he acquiesced. "I just couldn't turn him down, knowing his own track record." Charlie Gardner spent fourteen years working as a volunteer with the Lights, and said he never regretted a moment of it.

Brent Foster, coach of the Canadian Men's Wheelchair Basketball Team at the 1992 Barcelona Olympics, believes "the whole idea just took off" after Gary got the first board of directors together. That group gave it the needed credibility and public profile. Subsequent fund-raising was successful enough that people could be hired to run the organization. And money was available for travel, an essential activity if there was any hope of getting more competition and upgrading the level of the athletes' performance.

Reg McClellan and Gary McPherson made a dynamic pair: Reg as the first coach who also played and Gary as the promoter and organizer. Reg appreciated Gary's abilities in looking after such things as logistics for the team, but he regarded as even more important Gary's rapport with players, coaches and board members, including knowledge of their personal lives. "For him, we were all an extended family," he said.

From that moment the team acquired a cohesiveness. True, there were fine players, even outstanding ones, but they had been "floundering around" without any real organization where they felt they belonged. Several struggled with poor self-esteem, partly from personal problems they couldn't shake. Ron Minor, who was destined to become a wheelchair player of international stature on a par with Rick Hansen, had had his trouble with the law. He and some buddies broke into a store in a southern Alberta town, and Ron was apprehended the very next day: his crutch marks in the snow gave him away.

When Ron was invited to Edmonton to join the team, he went all out for the game. Almost penniless, he didn't even have a wheelchair. Reg found Ron Minor willing to make a commitment to wheelchair basketball like few others. And in due course he became a champion. For Ron, the sport was a springboard to a new life.

When Braden Hirsch first came to Edmonton from Saskatoon to play wheelchair basketball, he couldn't believe how "a bunch of fit, muscular athletic guys would gather around a pale, sickly-looking guy in a wheelchair." At age nineteen he had been thrown from an out-of-control car and suffered a spinal injury with permanent paralysis of his legs. He subsequently learned the game and played at a recreational level in

Saskatoon, but he wanted to play more competitively and he welcomed the opportunity to come to Edmonton to join the Lights.

As the organization grew, Gary spent more time on the phone looking for help. Janet Ross, of slow-pitch fame, worked in Gary's office at the Aberhart, doing all kinds of office work and escorting Gary to numerous meetings. Darlene Steljes, respiratory therapist from the Aberhart, often accompanied the team on their travels, looking after equipment and wheelchairs. Widowed as a young woman a few years before, she said the Northern Lights became "my social life."

When Braden Hirsch arrived, he found what he called "a first-class organization" and a so-so team that seemed to show potential. The players moved fast, wheeling their chairs up and down and around the basketball court with amazing speed and agility, but they lacked scoring punch. They won a few games, but repeatedly lost to the BC squad that bore the peculiar name of the Vancouver Cable Cars. Braden found it was no cinch getting on the team: more than thirty wheelchair athletes were vying for a position. They played at the ACT Centre, a wonderful facility especially designed to accommodate persons with physical disabilities, where Bob Steadward and Gary served on an advisory committee to the builders.

A year or so later the Lights began to gel, and thereafter there was no looking back. They beat their archrivals, the Vancouver Cable Cars, ending their dominance once and for all.

Then they were on a roll. They beat the Ontario team by forty-five points in the final game for the Canadian championships, and went on to win the Canadian title seven years in a row. Then in the early 1980s they started competing with American teams, playing in the Challenge Cup circuit. At one time they were ranked as high as number two in North America. A team from California that they had beaten twice consistently held the number-one spot. In international competitions, eight of the twelve players on Canada's national team were members of the Northern Lights.

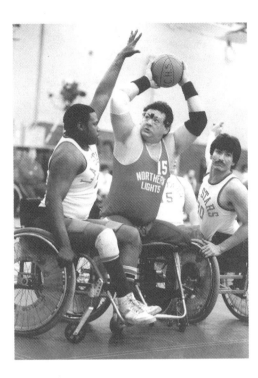

"Muscling in": John Belanger of the Northern Lights holds the ball in a tight competition against the Los Angeles Stars at the Northwest Regional Basketball Tournament in June, 1981.

Edmonton Journal

Soon the sporting public was hearing about this team that seemed to have come out of nowhere. A twenty-one-year-old sports columnist writing for the *Edmonton Journal* and the *Spokesman* decided to cover wheelchair sports. Disabled by cerebral palsy since birth, Cam Tait was already a much-respected reporter who had been on the phone to Gary McPherson. They became good friends. "I'm probably the forty-seventh person to tell you he's a wonderful man," Cam once said. He was entranced with the speed and finesse of wheelchair basketball, but even more impressed with the zest for life it seemed to give the disabled athletes. Thanks primarily to Cam Tait, the Northern Lights were brought into the public eye. Later Cam found himself "travelling all over North America with the team" and reporting back to the *Edmonton Journal*.

Cam remembers one occasion when players and coaches were lounging in a restaurant after a game—some on crutches, some amputees, some

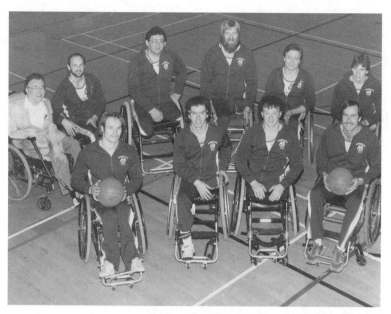

The 1985 Alberta Northern Lights Wheelchair Basketball Team, with General Manager Gary McPherson.

polio survivors with braces, and some with wheelchairs. With a puzzled look on his face, a man in the restaurant walked up, surveyed the bunch of muscular athletes and asked, "Are you some sort of sports team or something?"

"Yeah, basketball," said one of the fellows.

"Holy mackerel!" was the answer. "You must have been in a pretty tough battle." Everyone in the restaurant roared with laughter.

Cam Tait was once asked which was the most exciting sporting event he ever covered. He answered right away: "That game in Eugene, Oregon."

In 1985, sixteen teams from cities in North America had come together in Eugene to compete for the Challenge Cup, emblematic of the best in wheelchair basketball. The team winning all four of its games in Eugene would go to Lexington, Kentucky, to play in the finals. The Northern Lights knew they were underdogs, but they wheeled, passed and shot like a fired-up championship team.

Under the skillful coaching of Brent Patterson, they won three successive games and found themselves in the semifinals against the Casa Colina Condors from Pomona, California, perpetual champions with a record of ninety-nine wins in a row. The Northern Lights knew they would have to dig deep, to play like they never had before, to play their hearts out.

It was close, oh, so close—a real barn-burner.

In the dying moments of the game, Ron Minor saw Randy Wyness whipping down the court and flipped a pass to him. Randy tossed the ball up and scored, putting the Lights two points up. Then the other team got a basket, tying the score as the buzzer sounded. A five-minute overtime followed, and the Condors quickly scored. The Lights controlled the ball thereafter but still ended up two points down as the five minutes was drawing to a close. Someone tossed the ball to Ron, a "clutch" player if ever there was one, and he popped it up and in, tying the score again.

Then came the second five-minute overtime. The Condors attacked, but Ron intercepted a pass, wheeled down and scored. The Lights scored again. Then they passed the ball around as a defensive ploy, until one of the opponents got fouled. The Lights made a substitution, bringing in a player with a reputation of accuracy from the foul line—a legitimate and clever move. He didn't miss, and the Lights won the game by ten points, becoming the first Canadian team to go to the finals. They lost out at Lexington, but it didn't seem to matter; at Eugene they had shown what they could do. It was truly their finest hour.

The game in Eugene had an interesting sequel. Weary but elated, the Lights were on the bus heading for Vancouver, where they would catch a plane home. While passing through a little town near Bellingham, Washington, they decided to stop. Gary knew that his friend Rick Hansen was staying there, one of the early stops on the first leg of his round-the-world Man in Motion tour. Rick was a star with the Vancouver Cable Cars, friendly rivals of the Northern Lights.

"Let's wake Rick up," someone suggested. They did just that. In a bleary-eyed state at 5:00 A.M., he got up and shook the hand of each player. "I was feeling kind of low, and it meant a lot that these sporting colleagues would stop and share their celebration with me," Rick said later.

Gary was "the driving force behind the whole [Northern Lights] program," Rick maintained. Gary showed incredible strength in building and maintaining a superb organization. Jack Donohue, former head coach of Canada's national men's basketball team of able-bodied players, gave Gary most of the credit for the resurgence of wheelchair basketball. "He believed in it passionately and had the knack of hauling people in. He's a nagger, but a good one."

Gary himself believes that the real success of the Northern Lights was not on the basketball court. At the beginning, many or most of the disabled players were leading aimless lives. They ended up being useful citizens, working at productive jobs or going to school. Randy Wyness, Ron Minor, Braden Hirsch and others could all tell you how their lives were changed.

17 | **Rick Hansen and the Man in Motion Tour**

GARY MCPHERSON AND RICK HANSEN first met in 1976 at the Canadian Games for the Physically Disabled in Cambridge, Ontario. In the future their paths would cross frequently, culminating in a solid and lasting friendship.

Hailing from Williams Lake, British Columbia, Rick had been an all-star athlete in school, playing and usually winning in everything from volleyball to basketball to pole-vaulting. But an accident in June 1973, when he was just fifteen, wrecked a potentially bright career in sports. He and a friend had hitched a ride in the back of a pickup truck whose driver lost control and hit the ditch. Rick was flung into the air and hit the rocky ground with a thud. When he tried to get up afterwards, his legs felt dead and would not move. His spinal cord had been severed.[1]

In the months that followed, Rick's life hit bottom. Gradually he inched his way out of an abyss of dejection and a feeling of worthlessness to the level ground of adaptation and hope. He completed high school and with the help of his coach, Bob Redford, decided that he need not give up his love for sports after all; he could get into wheelchair sports. He quickly learned that "those guys are tough athletes."

He attended the University of British Columbia and graduated, becoming the first disabled person to get a degree in physical education.[2]

He joined the Vancouver Cable Cars wheelchair basketball team, where he played with a young fellow called Terry Fox from Simon Fraser University. Both he and Terry, who had undergone high amputation of his leg for bone cancer, starred for the Cable Cars, who won five national championships in six years.

There seemed to be no limit to Rick's accomplishments in wheelchair sports. In 1979, he played wheelchair basketball in the world championships at Tampa, Florida, with the Canadian national men's team, a team managed by Gary McPherson. In Gary's opinion, Rick Hansen and Ron Minor were, in addition to being tops on the basketball court, two of the world's best wheelchair track athletes. In 1982, Rick won nine gold medals at the Pan-American Wheelchair Games in Halifax. Later that year he was named, along with Wayne Gretzky, Canada's outstanding athlete of the year.

But Rick was aiming elsewhere. In 1981, he had noticed the impact of Terry Fox's attempt to run across Canada to raise money for cancer research. He was a friend and admirer of Terry, whose monumental effort to walk endless miles on an artificial leg inspired Rick to do something equally adventurous and unusual, but different. "I was always looking for my next journey."

Long before Terry's heroic endeavour, he had dreamed about wheeling around the world. He would set out on such an adventure with certain goals: to raise money for research into and rehabilitation of spinal cord injuries, to enhance the profile of wheelchair sport and to somehow change the way society looks at people with disabilities. He would push his wheelchair around the world. The year was 1985.

He could count on his family to help. Stan Stronge, coach of the Vancouver Cable Cars and a builder *par excellence* of sports for the disabled, and Gary McPherson, a friend, promoter and manager of wheelchair games, were both there to join in the planning and organizing of the Man in Motion tour. A crucial initial move was to get the endorsement and support of two important organizations working for the disabled: the Canadian Paraplegic Association (CPA) and the Canadian Wheelchair

Sports Association (CWSA). At a special meeting of the CWSA board, Executive-director Dean Mellway and President Gary McPherson did their utmost to get the members behind Rick's ambitious project.

"Are you serious? Rolling your wheelchair around the world?" many of them asked. In the end, however, they all gave their assent. The BC Paraplegic Foundation lent moral and financial support. Standing on this firm base, Rick and his team could then approach business firms for sponsorship. Almost fifty sponsors, corporate and individual, came through, some just a little dubious about Rick's "wild scheme."

On March 21, 1985, in the presence of the parents of his late friend Terry Fox and BC Premier Bill Bennett, Rick Hansen embarked on his round-the-world tour. He set out from Vancouver with an entourage of bikers, walkers, sign bearers and a motorhome emblazoned with the Man in Motion logo.

Over a period of two years, he rolled his wheelchair through thirty-four countries, up mountain roads and along seaside trails, through dust in Portugal and snow in northern Ontario, along lonely stretches of flat prairie and through the centre of big cities like Paris, San Francisco and Moscow. In Rome he was received by Pope John Paul II, and in Ottawa he was greeted by Prime Minister Brian Mulroney, who gave him a cheque for one million dollars. This large donation from the federal government helped to get the Canadian people behind the Man in Motion tour.

He needed that cheque. Arriving back in Newfoundland in August 1986, after racking up over thirty-two thousand kilometres (20,000 miles), the tour's trust fund held only two hundred thousand dollars. Rick wasn't bitter, just a little disappointed. Even so, despite his fatigued state, he felt a warm glow of optimism that his fellow Canadians would rally around. His optimism was justified: by the time he reached southern Ontario, the trust fund had climbed to three million dollars, and when he arrived at the Saskatchewan/Alberta border in late February 1987, it had hit the six-million-dollar mark.

The Alberta committee for the Man in Motion tour had been meeting for the previous eight months. Reg McClellan, founder of the Northern

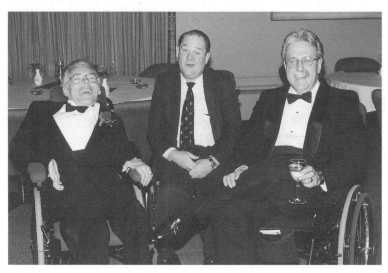

Gary McPherson and Vance Milligan, co-chairmen of the Alberta Man in Motion Committee celebrate with Cam Tait of the Edmonton Journal.

Janet Tkachyk

Lights, could think of no one more competent than Gary McPherson to work as chairman. Reg put forward his name. It would be a hefty undertaking for a fellow already busy enough with wheelchair basketball and the likes, but Gary consented. Eric Boyd, working with the Alberta division of the Canadian Paraplegic Association, agreed to co-chair. Both knew, respected and admired Rick Hansen, and wanted to do the best they could for him. Vance Milligan, a paraplegic lawyer from Calgary, agreed to co-chair the plans for the southern part of the province. Gary calls Vance "a wonderful organizer with contacts like you wouldn't believe."

Gary was fortunate in having the help of Leona Holland, a capable administrator who had been working with Bob Steadward and who excelled at rallying volunteers. They got valuable help from the Man in Motion head office in Vancouver in terms of fund-raising and media relations. They also learned how to avoid some of the "mistakes" made in Ontario and Manitoba. But the head office was quick to assure them to feel free to be flexible and original.

One day in August, Gary sat down, applied his considerable capacity for envisaging and planning, then got a helper to make a list of tasks. First, they'd have to organize a committee of people from the community. They had only eight months to raise funds for the project and solicit the help of volunteers, thousands of them if possible, from all over the province. There would be the inevitable administration, accounting and organizing of meetings. To get the participation of every possible Albertan, they would have to consult with business people, schools, municipalities, provincial government departments and as many media outlets as possible.

The campaign preparing for the arrival of the Man in Motion tour in Alberta rapidly gained momentum. Forty-three community committees were actively involved in supporting Rick Hansen when he arrived. In remote Fort McMurray, Gary's sister Kim and her husband, Roger, arranged a successful cross-country skiing relay that raised fourteen thousand dollars for Rick. Competition between the two committees in Edmonton and Calgary intensified with sizzling phone messages between Vance and Gary: "Say, can you beat this?" or "Guess what we're gonna do when he comes?" The traditional Edmonton/Calgary rivalry took on a new twist. Ideas simply flew.

Then Premier Don Getty announced that the government would match, dollar for dollar, all private donations, and the whole ambitious program shifted into high gear. Alberta Government Telephones (AGT) provided free communication between Rick's party, wherever they happened to be, and various regional committees, especially those in Calgary and Edmonton. The RCMP assigned a constable to escort the tour all the way through Alberta.

February 23, 1987, was a cloudy day at the Alberta/Saskatchewan border just west of Maple Creek. At a point on the Trans-Canada Highway, a crowd of people including Premier Getty and the mayor of Medicine Hat had assembled on a portable stage decorated with flags and signs to welcome Rick and his entourage to Alberta. Gary and some of his co-workers had driven down from Edmonton for the occasion; it was his responsibility to introduce all the honoured guests. He was not surprised to find his old friend Rick bone-weary but thankful to be in Alberta and nearing the end of his 40,072 kilometre (24,900 mile) journey.

The route across the province had been measured off in kilometres, and anyone wanting to "buy" a kilometre for Rick for one hundred dollars could put up a sign bearing his or her name. At kilometre 4, Rick saw the name of Reg McClellan, his former wheelchair basketball opponent who wore jersey number 4; at kilometre 99, he wasn't surprised to see the name of Wayne Gretzky.

During his twenty-eight days of wheeling through to Calgary, Edmonton and then west to the BC border, Rick travelled as a celebrity, often escorted by cyclists and other wheelchair athletes, and greeted by cheering people all along the way. Wherever he stopped, he found himself in front of a thicket of TV cameras, tape recorders and reporters with notepads. The media considered the whole tour a fascinating news story, not just a project. Cam Tait covered the entire Alberta leg for the *Edmonton Journal*. Just about every community had concocted a project to give Rick financial support.

Vance Milligan, an unwilling captain at the start, soon found himself up to his eyebrows in Man in Motion schemes, and he virtually gave up his job to serve as chairman of the Calgary committee, coordinating a multitude of activities. In his mind, Rick's courage and perseverance, to say nothing of his worthy goals, were greatly inspiring, and Vance was determined to make the Alberta portion of the tour a top-notch event. His phone rang constantly, often with several calls a day from his Edmonton counterpart.

But more often than not, people wanted to know where to make donations and volunteer to help. One phone call came from Eaton's department store, inviting Vance to come down and collect a cheque: the employees had staged their own wheelchair race right in the store and collected a sizeable amount from bets and donations.

When Rick arrived in Calgary, a crowd of nine thousand awaited at the Saddledome to welcome him, including Mayor Ralph Klein and other noteworthies. Part of the program was a "shoot-out" with Mayor Klein trying to fire pucks into the net from centre ice. Vance's committee had solicited puck sponsorships from several major companies: if Klein scored, the sponsors would turn over five thousand dollars for the "Score One for Rick" campaign; if he missed, they were stuck for only half that amount. When Klein missed with his first several shots, everyone groaned. Then he started to hit the mark and everyone cheered. He got lots of practice that night, firing twenty-one pucks all told.

Not to be outdone, Edmonton aimed to surpass Calgary and probably succeeded in ingenuity. There too Mayor Lawrence Decore did his best to score goals from centre ice, with the same amounts attending success or failure. Then Rick was allowed a shot, this time for ten thousand dollars. But he had never before shot a puck from his wheelchair, and even with Wayne Gretzky at his side cheering him on, he could not quite hit the net.

At Hobbema, near Edmonton, a huge crowd including members of four First Nations bands packed a gymnasium to show their appreciation of the Man in Motion. A tribal elder, overcome with tears, offered a prayer for Rick. Then came traditional dances in his honour, gifts of blankets and moccasins, and donations totalling twenty-three thousand dollars. At the end, Rick was made an honorary band member.

A few days later Rick was presented with a sort of memento, not a gift, that he would treasure for all his life.

At Edmonton's Northlands Coliseum a crowd of thousands, including the mayor and other dignitaries, had gathered at a reception to honour Rick. Charlie Gardner, then chairman of the board of the Northern Lights, sat alongside Gary McPherson, who had an old basketball jersey draped over the arm of his wheelchair. On the back was the name "Fox." Terry Fox and Rick Hansen had played as regulars for the Vancouver wheelchair basketball team, but at times they were loaned to the Northern

Lights for international competitions. Gary had kept Terry Fox's jersey in his clothes closet for several years.

During the course of the evening, Charlie Gardner pushed Gary's wheelchair onto the stage, where Gary told the audience about the jersey and asked Charlie to present it to Rick. Rick accepted it but could not speak, he was so overcome. Terry's run across Canada on his artificial leg had come to an end at Thunder Bay, Ontario, on September 1, 1980, when severe chest pain forced him to halt. His cancer had recurred, and he died on June 28, 1981.

Vance Milligan firmly believes that "more money was raised during that intensive twenty-eight-day period than in the history of fund-raising." At the end, a total of $5.2 million dollars was turned over to the Man in Motion trust fund, totalling almost as much as had been raised in all the provinces east of Alberta.

· · · · ·

WHAT WAS THE LEGACY of the Alberta tour? Knowing that Rick had some definite ideas to promote, Gary arranged a meeting at the Alberta legislature. The government put up a red-carpeted ramp for Rick, welcoming him in fine style. He outlined his goals before Premier Don Getty and seven of his cabinet ministers. Rick's original plan for the Man in Motion tour was not only to raise money but also to stimulate political decisions that would benefit the disabled community. Understandably, the government stipulated that the money it had matched be spent in Alberta.

The Alberta branch of the Canadian Paraplegic Association received generous support. Additionally, the Alberta Paraplegic Foundation was established with Vance Milligan as chair and Gary McPherson as vice-chair. The goals of the foundation were well-defined: to support rehabilitation of disabled people, to further research in the area of spinal cord injury, to promote wheelchair sports of all kinds and to build up awareness of the potential of people with disabilities.

The Rick Hansen Centre at the University of Alberta was later opened by Premier Getty. Founded by Dr. Bob Steadward, it had previously gone under the name of the Research and Training Centre for the Physically Disabled (now, it has become the Steadward Centre).

Both Rick and Gary wanted the government to inaugurate a program that would make buildings and facilities accessible to people in wheelchairs. They felt that an advisory council was needed to present to the government the overall needs and desires of the disability community.

As a result of that meeting in the legislature, Premier Getty committed the government to the formation of the Premier's Council on the Status of Persons with Disabilities. He appointed a steering committee that included two people recommended by Gary: Greg Latham and Eric Boyd, wheelchair athlete and executive with the Canadian Paraplegic Association. After extensive public consultation in which, among other things, services for the disabled were reviewed, the committee issued a report which ultimately resulted in legislation that created the council.

In effect, the Alberta leg of the Man in Motion tour began a series of events and changes in the lives of people with all kinds of disabilities, changes that would probably have taken years had it not been for the astounding feat of Rick Hansen and the great impact he made on the general public and governments. Gentleman that he is, Rick was quick to give credit for success to Gary McPherson and Vance Milligan, saying, "Those two did an amazing job." He spoke with conviction when he said, "That Gary is the most able guy I have ever met."

Rick Hansen still travels, but not around the world. At the Rick Hansen Institute on the campus of the University of British Columbia, he and his staff work hard to support research into spinal cord injuries and paralysis in centres located in Canada and overseas.

Rick's philosophy? "If we have our sails set so that the wind fills them, we'll move forward."

18 | Clayton, Wise and Gentle Friend

IF YOU ASK GARY about that notorious group on the polio ward called "the boys," he will freely admit that they were all brothers, brothers without blood ties. For long years they lived in close proximity, at the beginning almost in each other's pockets, sharing each other's lives on a rollercoaster of hope and disappointment, exultation and despair, tears and laughter. They were enterprising, lusty and even boisterous as a group. Being youths, they often said and did foolish things, but someone always hauled them back from the brink of disaster.

Clayton May was that someone.

Hit with polio in 1953 when he was twelve, Clayton May came up from the little town of Killam, Alberta. He was admitted to the Edmonton General Hospital before being transferred to the polio ward at the University Hospital. He was probably the most disabled of all the young fellows on Station 32, paralyzed from the neck down and, like Gary, unable to breathe. Without the iron lung, he would not have survived. Gradually he gained some control over his breathing, but he had to return to the iron lung at night. Then he learned frog-breathing, but apart from slight movement in one little finger, he never regained the use of his arms or legs.

Dissimilar in disposition, Clayton May and Gary McPherson become close buddies and kindred spirits. Clayton was a couple of years older, more mature and somewhat wiser in the ways of the world. They were like opposites that attract: Gary, the brash teenager with the loose and sometimes sharp tongue; Clayton, the quiet older brother, full of ideas but keeping himself carefully in check. The two irritated each other and frequently got into heated verbal battles, but the strife was short-lived and somehow served only to cement the bonds of brotherhood. And they got involved in all kinds of schemes and activities together.

His body may have been inert, but Clayton's mind was keen, always exploring new ideas and new things to learn. He and Bob Johnson saw no reason why they shouldn't become millionaires, or at least make a few dollars on the stock market or at the racetrack. In fact, the two of them were so captivated with horse-racing that they actually bought a racehorse—which failed to earn anything but heartache. Keen to learn Morse code with the rest of the would-be amateur radio operators in the late 1960s, Clayton took great delight in sending messages through a microswitch fitted to his teeth.

Gary remembers that Clayton had a great interest in life, following current events daily on radio and TV, and doing his best to keep informed. A custom-made device suspended from a bracketed arm attached to his bed and reaching down to his cheek enabled him, if he raised his head and touched it lightly, to turn on the TV. He loved reading, but needed the help of a volunteer to turn the pages.

Don Buchanan, former orthopedic patient and later a judge, called him a wonderful conversationalist, intellectually stimulating and interested in people's lives. Others described him as charming and witty. Not once could Gary or others among Clayton's friends and visitors remember him complaining or lamenting his fate. Occupational therapist Fran Osokin thought Clayton remarkable with his wise remarks and witticisms. "There never was a 'poor me' word from him," she said.

Respirology specialist Dr. Brian Sproule has good memories of the May-McPherson duo: "Gary, the hustler, and Clayton, the sage and steadying influence." Young Gary needed a mentor in those days, someone a little older and wiser to keep him from flying off into space or sinking into a pit. Clayton was the stable and inspiring friend who would help him along the way and teach him "lessons for life" that he would always treasure. He taught him to observe, think and reason. "While the others were raving and hollering, Clayton was listening quietly, nodding his head now and then," a hospital staff member said, "and finally offering his analysis of the whole issue (or whatever it was) and suggesting answers."

Clayton and Gary worked together as a team, serving as political agitators or spokesmen for the ward in times of need. Leadership of the patients seemed to fall naturally into their hands. Refusing to be treated like prisoners, they battled against hospital and nursing administration, demanding that restrictive rules and regulations be relaxed. Why shouldn't they be allowed to stay out after 9:00 P.M., they asked? Why should Clayton have to sign out in order to go visit his mother in Strome? You'd think he was a school kid, they complained. They won that battle hands-down, and the patients gained the freedom they merited as long-term residents. Gary and Clayton weren't worried about retribution. "They couldn't throw us out on the street."

Both patients and staff on the polio ward needed a sympathetic listener when times were tough or hurtful; in Clayton, they found someone who met their needs. Darlene Steljes had been through the valley of the shadow when her young husband died. She turned to Clayton, "someone more stable than ninety percent of our society" and found "restoration for my soul."

Of course, Clayton was far from being infallible, and his friends would never let him forget the time when he insisted on "following the book," ending in disaster when the mouth-watering roast pig was completely cremated. Generally, however, Clayton did the right thing.

It was through Clayton that Gary was "given" the finest gift of his life, a loving partner and wife. Clayton masterminded a New Year's Eve party for the Aberhart patients on December 31, 1980, and invited as many

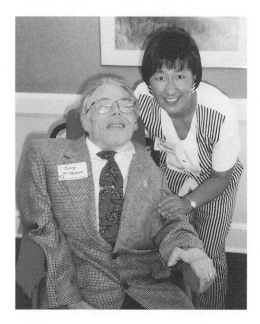

Gary McPherson and
Valerie Kamitomo.
Janet Tkachyk

single girls as he could round up. Among the guests were Val Kamitomo and her friend Diane Firby, whom Gary knew much better than Val. When the hour of midnight struck, Gary happened to be with Val, a soft-spoken, cheerful Japanese-Canadian woman originally from Raymond, Alberta.

Val had graduated with a B.Sc. in nursing from the University of Alberta in 1980 and was hired as a nurse at the Aberhart Hospital. She spent her first ten months on the polio ward but was not impressed one bit either by the ward or by Gary McPherson. "He was so intimidating and sort of bossy. He could easily embarrass a person and get away with it because he could produce a cute little smile that was hard to ignore." But Val herself was pretty good at repartee, and when probed about her racial origin, she blithely responded, "Eskimo, of course." At Clayton's party, Gary managed to produce that same smile before bestowing on her the traditional New Year's Eve kiss. Thereafter he became less intimidating. Although well aware that he might be accused of robbing the cradle (Val was twelve years his junior), he soon found out that Val was an exceptional person, an absolute rarity.

Unlike Gary, whose slow-pitch coaching and wheelchair basketball affairs took him far from hospital confines, Clayton left hospital only on rare occasions, and as the years passed, fewer visitors came to see him. Although by this time he and Gary occupied separate rooms at the Aberhart Hospital, Gary made a point of dropping in frequently to see his old friend.

Then one day in July, Clayton went into respiratory failure. He was taken to the intensive care unit, barely conscious, feverish and breathing in weak, shallow breaths. Clayton died on July 10, 1988, finally freed from hospital life after thirty-five years.

To say farewell to Clayton and celebrate his life, a convoy of vans and cars carrying patients, staff and friends travelled down to Strome for his funeral. "It was like losing a member of the family," nursing aide Lorraine Habekost said. At the funeral, Gary remembers having trouble breathing, such was the overwhelming emotion he felt for his dear friend. Judge Don Buchanan was there too and, like everyone else, sobbing unashamedly.

For many people, both able-bodied and polio-disabled, Clayton was a veritable Rock of Gibraltar. Somewhere deep within that feeble frame, a quiet source of strength sustained him during the long years and offered solace to others. As a boy Clayton had attended church with his parents, but like many adolescents—in and out of hospital—he had drifted away. But one suspects that his Creator did not desert him but blessed him with an enduring peace, quietness and courage.

Clayton has not been forgotten. At the Good Samaritan Millwoods Centre for Assisted Living in Edmonton, a crowd gathered some time later to dedicate a new extension called the Clayton May Court. Judge Don Buchanan spoke before a large assembly of the old polio crowd, wheelchair basketball players, friends and families. Don testified that Clayton had enriched his life, inspiring him to do better and enjoy life to the full.

In 2000, Gary published a book, *With Every Breath I Take*, and dedicated it to his friend:

For Clayton May—my friend, mentor, and confidant. He will forever live in my heart and be a part of me.

19 | Vacating Hospital for a Val-uable Alliance

"AFTER CLAYTON DIED, it was almost like I was getting permission to leave hospital," Gary said. For thirty-three years, Clayton and Gary had been soul mates in an institution that tends to be soul-destroying. During those long years of joys and sorrows, the ties that bound them together remained strong. "There was nobody I cared for quite as much as Clayton," Gary said several times. "We were like brothers."

Up until 1973, they had been together with six to eight others in one large ward that almost demanded collective living. After moving into the Aberhart Hospital with its two- and four-bedded rooms, each patient was freer to develop his own interests and activities, his own individuality. The two friends mingled less frequently. Gary used the hospital as a "base of operations"—his frequent out-of-hospital jaunts with the Canadian Wheelchair Sports Association (CWSA), slow-pitch coaching and the Man in Motion tour came in the way of their fellowship. "I always felt bad leaving Clayton behind," Gary said.

The hospital was home, but things were changing. While Clayton's death severed one emotional attachment, another was slowly gaining momentum. One day it would burst into bloom, like the bud of a calypso orchid.

After their first encounter on New Year's Eve, 1980, Val and Gary started going out together—to sports events, dinner, and social parties. One of the orderlies from the Aberhart would always accompany them, not as a chaperone but to lift Gary into or out of the wheelchair.

Gary refused to allow petite Val, who was only 150 centimeters (4'11") tall, to drive the van, thinking she couldn't reach the foot pedals. That proved to be the first of several slight disagreements in which she proved him wrong. Occasionally he would go to her home for supper. He found her a bright companion, "fun to be with," but stopped there in his thinking about her.

After three to four years of casual contact, often separated by long periods of silence, Val announced in no uncertain terms that she was going to break up with him. She meant business; he just hadn't been paying her enough attention. Gary was shattered—the news literally took his breath away. He realized he'd been pretty heartless.

Probably the institutional mindset had stultified his social growth, in particular his relationship with girls. In our society where males usually take the initiative, Gary felt at a loss, having to rely entirely on words and expressions. As an adolescent, he lusted after a pretty girl like all the rest of "the boys." Disability had not stifled all the feelings, emotions and urges.

Later, as a man of twenty-seven, he realized that his relationship with women needed some refinement and finesse. And it would show improvement as he began to better understand his own self-image and what he had to offer as a person. It's not that women weren't attracted to Gary. Lorraine Habekost remembers that girls were "always hanging around him, he had such a warm personality." Asked to explain the reason, her husband Norman quipped, "Some girls go for the brain instead of the body."

It took a life-threatening lung hemorrhage to bring Val and Gary together again. Without warning, one day Gary began to cough up large amounts of bright red blood. The bleeding stopped spontaneously, only to recur next day. Alarmed that he might drown in his own blood, doctors took him to the intensive care unit, inserted a bronchoscope down his windpipe and put pressure on the affected point to control the bleeding. Val's friend Diane, who worked at the Aberhart at that time, heard of the dangerous hemorrhage and called her to come over.

"It just tore at my heart strings to see him in such danger," said Val. Finally they both realized how much they meant to each other. But neither one wanted to do things in a hurry, and another six years passed before they got married.

During those years Gary began to realize how unique was the bright, little Japanese-Canadian woman who cared so much for him. Years before, Val had turned down a date with a disabled fellow because the whole idea of going out with such a person embarrassed her. When she encountered the boisterous, irrepressible gang on the polio ward, she had to reassess her whole attitude, though it took Gary to revolutionize her feelings about the disabled. "I didn't really look upon him as handicapped, knowing his other great qualities," she said. "I saw him more as a person."

But marrying a quadriplegic was another matter. She knew well enough the anguish that Liz Baril had endured when she married Henri and tried to care for him at home without any help. When children arrived, the stresses and strains became unbearable. Val's mother tried not to express her deep concern over the hazard-strewn journey Val might be embarking on, but the worries were there. Val's nursing experience would stand her in good stead, but would it be enough?

The practicalities of moving out of hospital deterred Gary. He had little income. The Northern Lights, whom he had served for some time on a volunteer basis, now paid him a modest salary. He got a part-time job at the Rick Hansen Centre as assistant director to Dr. Bob Steadward, but he determined not to leave the hospital until the proper supports, such as home care, were in place. The "Polio Program" legislation had been passed, but he would have to go on a waiting list, like everyone else. In due course he would qualify for the self-managed program, which provides a sum of money each month and allows the recipient to hire the help needed.

No admirer of the institutional life, he nevertheless felt that leaving the Aberhart Hospital would be like walking out on a cracking limb. Over the years all his practical needs had been met so completely. Vance Milligan, his committee co-chair for the Man in Motion tour, regarded Gary's move to leave hospital as courageous, especially since his life was so much at risk. But he believed that "it was necessary for his growth and development to take that step."

Equally frightening was another thought: suppose marriage to Val should fail? Foreseeing that unlikely but possible outcome, Gary planned to keep the umbilical cord to the hospital intact until the year after their wedding.

What helped Gary through the swamp of uncertainty was not a sudden surge of resolve but a lesson he had learned from an older patient back on Station 67. A man in his late sixties, Mr. Hack suffered from a severe and painful kyphosis (hunchback deformity) which sharply restricted his activity. His wife of more than forty years was always there, catering to his needs and providing companionship in his loneliness. He just couldn't find enough nice things to say about her, but one day he confided to Gary that it had not always been so.

"When we got married, I really didn't love her much," he said, "but I grew to love her." Mr. Hack's life soon came to an end, but that brief conversation with Gary had a deep impact. He hadn't fallen head over heels in love with Val, admitting that theirs was more of a friendship "with a relationship more of the head than the heart." But all along he had somehow sensed the potential of their relationship. Like Mr. Hack, he would do his best to appreciate his new partner and grow to love her.

Gary finally slipped a ring on Val's finger in December 1987, but true to form, feelings of uncertainty still raced through his mind. First, there was the doubt about the outcome, and second, the feeling that he would be deserting his old friend Clayton. It was a beautiful ring of diamonds and sapphires, but he denied it was a symbol of engagement, insisting on calling it a "friendship ring."

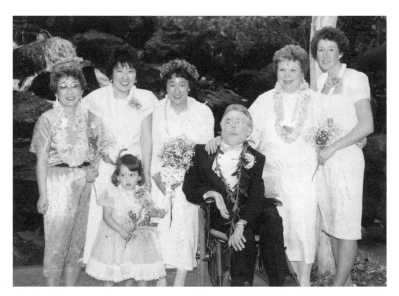

The wedding party in Honolulu, Hawaii. From left to right: Val's mother Katie, her sister Elaine, little Kerby the flower girl, Val and Gary, Gary's mother Dorothy , and "best man" Janet Ross. Janet Tkachyk (nee Ross)

Gary finally decided to marry Val. Their wedding would involve a modest ceremony in Hawaii, in Gary's mind a heaven-on-earth spot. Hawaii still held for him wonderful memories from 1976, when he had organized the holiday for thirty-one patients and staff from the polio ward. But who would they choose for best man?

Early in December 1988, he asked their dear friend Janet Ross out for coffee. Janet had been an enthusiastic player on the Bad News AIRS slow-pitch team and a faithful volunteer worker during the Man in Motion tour in 1987. Both Gary and Val considered Janet as "solid as a rock." She pushed Gary's wheelchair down Whyte Avenue to a coffee shop, both talking about everything else but the topic burning in Gary's brain. But while they drank coffee together that morning, unshakeable Janet broke down in tears of joy when Gary asked her to be the best man at their wedding. Janet was unaware that a woman could fill that role, but that in itself was not so disruptive. She was emotionally overcome, knowing

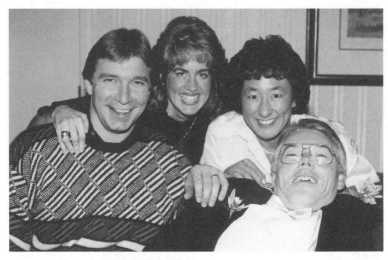

Rick and Amanda Hansen joined Valerie and Gary McPherson at the newly-weds' reception, held in Edmonton in February, 1989.

about the vast number of Gary's friends across the land, so many of whom had been important in his life. Yet he chose her.

Everything was kept low-key, almost secretive. They invited their respective mothers to accompany them to Hawaii for a holiday. Not until they were airborne did the mothers find out that there would be a wedding too. Val's aunt and her sister Elaine, who would serve as maid of honour, were also invited. Plans were made to meet Val's sister and brother-in-law, living in Australia, in Hawaii. Ever the meticulous planner, Gary had requested a friend in Honolulu to lay plans for hotel accommodation and a justice of the peace to carry out the ceremony. His old friend Cheryl Lavoie, who had been so helpful in 1976, arranged for the party to be picked up at the airport in a limousine.

On New Year's Eve 1988, the eighth anniversary of their first date, Val and Gary stood in front of a simulated waterfall in Honolulu's Hilton hotel and became husband and wife. Janet calls that day one of the high-lights of her life, just to see these two dear friends finally together.

Among the twenty-one participants and guests were Cheryl Lavoie and Beth Myers, a former nurse on the polio ward, now living in Hawaii.

Gary knew that his friend Don Getty and his wife would be in Hawaii on holiday at the time, and he invited them to attend. Don and Margaret walked over to the wedding from the condo where they were staying. "It was wonderful to be there," he said.

Gary and Val were married in the type of quiet, simple ceremony they wanted. Returning to Edmonton, they found that Bob Steadward had laid plans for a gala post-wedding reception, a dress-up affair at a downtown hotel. Crowds of friends, some using wheelchairs but most able-bodied and walking around, cheered and drank toasts to the happiness of an extra-ordinary couple.

Has it been a happy marriage? Asked for her opinion ten years later, Val replied without hesitation, "Oh yeah, excellent! Never a dull moment."

20 | Premier's Council

BEFORE RICK HANSEN LEFT ALBERTA in his wheelchair to conclude his Man in Motion world tour, he and Gary had obtained the commitment of Premier Don Getty's government to establish the Premier's Council on the Status of Persons with Disabilities.

To work out the role and function of such a council, Gary had recommended the formation of a steering committee that would include Greg Latham, as chairman, and Eric Boyd. Previously employed by the City of Edmonton's Transportation Planning Branch, Greg had worked with Gary on a project called the Disabled Adult Transportation System. After extensive public consultations in which, among other things, the services for the disabled were reviewed, the committee issued a report which ultimately resulted in legislation that created the council.

But the public consultations didn't always run smoothly. Greg chaired one meeting attended by about three hundred people, including a smattering of city councillors and the press and TV cameras. A copy of the committee's proposals was distributed to the assembly. To his horror, Greg saw one man stand up in the front row, mutter a few unintelligible words and then throw the document on the floor. Greg breathed a little easier when he realized a moment later that the fellow had cerebral palsy and had inadvertently dropped the paper.

In 1988, the Premier's Council on the Status of Persons with Disabilities came into being. It was given a ten-year mandate to listen to, cooperate with and facilitate the work of more than six hundred organizations serving people with disabilities. With a maximum of fifteen members, some disabled and some not, but all interested in the field of disability, the council would serve as an advisory group to the government, reporting directly to cabinet.

The Alberta Premier's Council was the second to be established in Canada, the first having been created in New Brunswick in 1983 as a result of the International Year of Disabled Persons. It required Rick Hansen's high profile and personal crusading to get one going in Alberta. And it's doubtful if the council would ever have come into being without the support of Premier Getty.

Don Getty sincerely wanted a group that would help the government in building awareness and developing the capacity to deal with disabled people and to promote the idea they are people with abilities. A former professional athlete himself, he stated that most of the disabled athletes he knew excelled in "mental toughness, determination and tenacity, far beyond what I had seen in other athletes and sports figures."

One evening in March 1988, Gary McPherson, still a patient of sorts at the Aberhart Hospital, received a phone call that would profoundly affect his lifestyle and career for the next ten years. It was Premier Don Getty calling: would Gary consider the job of chairman of the newly created Premier's Council?

Gary slept fitfully that night. But living with challenges as his daily bread, he could hardly turn away from this one. By April 1, he was grooming himself for the job, and the next month an office was set up for him. Gary had great hopes that Eric Boyd would come onboard as executive-director, feeling that "few people anywhere have a better understanding of the problems and needs of the disabled," but Eric demurred.

Finally, on the last day for receiving applications, Eric applied and was accepted. Another council member was Wendy Buckley, who became senior administrative assistant and stayed on for eight years.

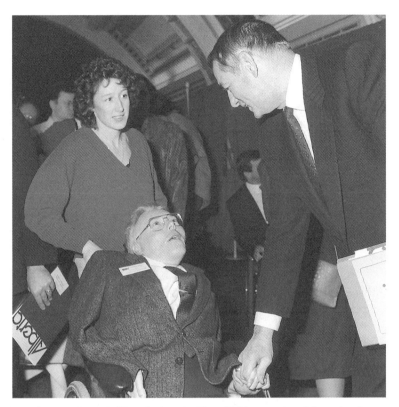

Premier Don Getty shaking the hand of Gary McPherson. Janet Ross stands behind Gary. Janet Tkachyk

Gary held no illusions that the job would be simple and uncompli-cated. But he felt that in his leadership capacity as a severely disabled person, he was in a unique position. Few disabled persons had been involved in decision-making processes, and almost none were working proactively. The council would be free to operate without government intervention, but it would certainly be at the beck and call of the disabled community. He anticipated that the pressure from the latter would be considerable.

Because the disabled communities had lacked cohesiveness, advo-cacy on their behalf would be a formidable challenge. Gary saw the need for a radical change in philosophy: simply maintaining people with disabilities and allowing them to exist was not enough; they needed to be liberated and allowed to function to their full capacity in the community.

As council chair, Gary would have responsibilities in many areas. First would be the hiring of staff and consultants, and building a profile for the new organization. He'd had lots of experience chairing meetings but less in preparing reports for the government. Building a network and liaison among disability groups would be high priority. And of course, the council would be responsible for developing policies and programs. Gary was not lacking in administrative skills, but he would need a strong team with vision and dedication.

For the first year of his tenure Gary lived at the Aberhart, working only half-time with the council. Then he gave up his job at the Rick Hansen Centre and became full-time chairman of the council. Eric Boyd worked cheek-by-jowl with Gary for six years, with Eric calling them "a strong team that worked very well together."

The council had a board of fifteen volunteers and a six-person secretariat to run the office. Eric managed most of the council business, while Gary served as the contact man between the secretariat and the volunteers, and as liaison man with government. After a year of operation, Eric hired Fran Vargo as a policy researcher.

It was a frightening proposition at the beginning—to be faced with a plethora of disability issues brought forward by the steering committee and the consultants hired for that purpose. Finally the council decided to categorize the various issues into community, employment, training and education, transportation, and so on. It wouldn't matter whether the disabled people were blind, suffering from multiple sclerosis or cerebral palsy, those categories still applied.

Then they circulated a questionnaire. When answers returned, the number-one concern—getting a seventy-percent rating—was the desire of disabled people to live in the community, not in an institution. Employment and education followed next in terms of priority. The needs were really no different from those of able-bodied people. It soon became clear that the focus should not be on the issue of disability and a medical diagnosis, but on the issue of need. If the needs were met, the disability would sink into the shadows.

One of the new council's first projects was building on the "Culture of Ability" paper produced by the Easter Seals organization to produce a document that would provide the framework for the government to create policy and programs. Four principles were to be articulated in that document: the value and worth of the individual; the right of persons to be consulted on issues that affect them; the right and responsibility of persons to be involved in the community; and the right of the person to make his or her own decisions, even if such decisions might be risky.

The action plan was a complicated blueprint including more than one hundred recommendations that involved some twenty-two government programs pertaining to people with disabilities. It was managed by Eric Boyd on behalf of the council after extensive consultation with disabled people and their advocates and families. It was important not only to transform public policy but also to change attitudes. The work done by Eric Boyd, Fran Vargo and Gary created a heightened sensitivity among government officials to issues affecting disabled people. As Gary said, the Premier's Council "certainly had an effect on the mentality of government."

In 1998, after ten years of service, Gary resigned as chairman of the Premier's Council. The council had been given a ten-year mandate, and he was willing to stay on for the duration, while feeling somewhat restless during the last couple of years. He had never before been involved in any activity for that long. As in his other activities, he liked to initiate various enterprises, then withdraw when momentum was assured. "I was more excited by the creation than by the maintenance," he said. Of course, the steady income was a great boon to his security, and he now had a family to take care of.

In some ways, it had been an extremely rewarding time for him; in other ways, not so. Asked whether the council accomplished its goals, he shook his head. But when asked for his opinion on whether the council's efforts improved the way people with disabilities live in Alberta, he answered, "We sure did."

Many disabled kids now attended public schools, a striking contrast to past years—when Gary had applied for school entrance as a teenager, he was rejected. There were plenty of Cam Taits, Percy Wickhams and Rick Hansens around. Gary remembers going to a bar once with his slow-pitch team and being rebuffed. At the time it hurt, but later he understood: "They were embarrassed to have me there." He believed it would not happen again. Nowadays people disabled from injury can expect rehabilitation, education, assistance with transportation and training to earn a living. Further, Greg Latham was adamant that "wheelchair access and transportation for the disabled in Edmonton is far ahead of any other place in Canada."

Janet Ross worked as Gary's personal attendant during part of his time with the council, and she often stayed with him during the many meetings he conducted. She was constantly amazed at his ability to get through an agenda and remember what had transpired, without being able to write a word. "He was fair and democratic," she said, "always careful what he said and diplomatic so as not to offend people's sensitivities."

Yet Gary received his share of criticism, sometimes overtly expressed, more often indirect or underhanded. He was accused of being "lazy, manipulative and abusive of his position." Was this harsh criticism justified? Eric Boyd, working as executive-director, thought not, and said he wanted to hear no such subversive rumblings, whether or not they had a basis in truth. Fortunately, such differences did not interfere with the good and effective work of the council over the ten-year period.

In the latter years of his role on the council, Gary encountered one frustration after another. The early 1990s became a time of extensive cutbacks by the Alberta government; as a result disability issues and programs suffered. A further source of disappointment was the indifference of the bureaucracy; as government priorities shifted, departments became less supportive of the council's mission. The creation of the

Alberta Economic Development Authority in 1994 suggested that the government was now giving priority to economic concerns. The social development agenda that included disability issues seemed to get sidelined.

The August 1998 issue of *Status Report*, the Premier's Council's quarterly newsletter on disability issues, reported Gary's impending departure from the council. It wasn't a time for retiring, but rather a change of ministry—Gary was moving to the university as special lecturer and adviser on issues involving people with disabilities. Premier Ralph Klein paid tribute to Gary's record: "Gary's service and dedication on behalf of people with disabilities is greatly appreciated by all Albertans. He has made many significant contributions over the last decade."[1]

Did Gary McPherson leave a worthwhile legacy after his ten years with the council? Randy Dickinson, his counterpart in New Brunswick, said: "He brought reps from the various disability groups together and got them to put aside their separate agendas and work collectively. He saw the importance of educating government officials. He saw the need for the business community to create an environment that would offer more employment opportunities for the disabled."

Russell Carr, consultant to the Premier's Council in the area of policy making for several years, made some surprising comments about Gary, including, "I've long since failed to see his wheelchair and what it meant." With respect to Gary's contributions, he added: "Gary is a man ahead of his time. He sees health in a spiritual and social sense. He emphasizes the importance of hope, social connectedness and interdependence. His greatest contribution is in helping us to understand what real health is."

21 | A Great Family

LIKE MOST COUPLES, Val and Gary wanted to have children, one of the greatest joys this life affords. For all but infertile couples, this ordinarily poses no great difficulties. But if one of the would-be parents is a quadriplegic, what then? Val conceived, not once but twice, to their great joy. Their friend Don Getty called that achievement a miracle, "an absolute miracle."

On October 24, 1989, their daughter Keiko was born. Gary accompanied Val to the maternity ward, as did Janet Ross (now Tkatchyk), who pushed his wheelchair. Well known around the hospital, Gary was told by a smirking nurse, "You're on the wrong ward, Gary. Better get back where you belong." Janet had attended prenatal classes with them both, and she was a great comfort to Val during the prolonged labour and delivery. Gary said witnessing the birth of a child whose life he had helped to create was "an unbelievable experience." That deeply emotional time also engendered in him great respect for women who endure the pain of childbirth. Janet too was overcome by emotion, first when Keiko was born, and moments later, when the parents informed her that the newborn baby would be called Keiko Janet McPherson.

On April 25, 1991, Jamie Robert made his debut. In the eyes of both children, their dad is "normal"; for all of their young lives, he has used a

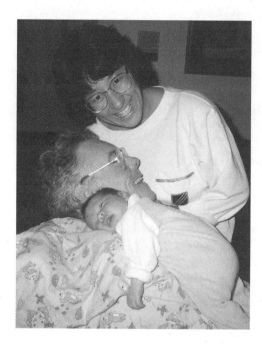

New family: Val, Gary and their daughter Keiko, only one month old.

Janet Tkachyk

wheelchair. They don't stare quizzically at other people in wheelchairs because the sight has been an everyday one for them. At one stage, however, when Keiko was still in kindergarten, she wanted to find out for sure what her dad could or could not do, and so she said, "Okay, Dad. It's time you got up and walked." She seemed content to be told that he couldn't.

Gary regrets that he was never able to bond with his children as babies, simply because he could not hold them in his arms. To make up for that, Val would hold them close to his face so he could kiss them. When the kids were small, Val felt unwilling to go out in the evening and leave them with their dad, insisting on having a baby-sitter. But as they grew older, they could do little things for him, and he did his best to interact with them by playing games and reading stories. And they quickly learned how to empty his "pee-bag," the rubber bag attached to his ankle that collects urine from a catheter draining his bladder.

Gary realized what a privilege it was for him to be a husband and father, a privilege he considered for most of his youth and adult life completely unattainable. He was determined to be "the best possible dad I could be, and to get away from my own little world of self-interest and help the kids with theirs." Having known one workaholic father who never really got to know his kids, Gary resolved to become a part of their lives insofar as his ability would permit. He and Val helped them with their homework, attended home-and-school meetings and rarely missed a soccer game when Keiko's team was playing. He did his best to set aside time for his children and always "tucked them into bed" at night.

Despite his physical state, Gary became an authority figure—not one to be feared, but one to be loved and respected. "They ignore me, just like most dads get ignored," he said, glad that his children relate to him as most kids do to their dads.

$$\cdot \quad \cdot \quad \cdot \quad \cdot \quad \cdot$$

TALKING PRIVATELY to Keiko and Jamie can be highly entertaining and informative, with no holds barred. At the time of the following conversation with the author, Keiko was nearly eleven and Jamie about nine.

"Were you at the university when your dad got the special degree?"

"Yeah. I had to wear an ugly, ugly jacket—the McPherson jacket or something. Mom made me wear it. It's gross," said Keiko.

"Do you play games with your dad?"

"Sometimes. At chess he cheats, trying to move his pawns all over. Then I have to remind him they can only move frontwards."

"Does he offer to help you with your homework?'

"Yes, but he doesn't really help much. When I tell him he's doing it wrong, he says, 'Don't criticize'."

"But you help your dad quite a lot, I bet. I've seen you feed him."

"Yeah, I do. But I usually eat some of his food. One spoonful for him, and one for me."

"What else do you do for him?"

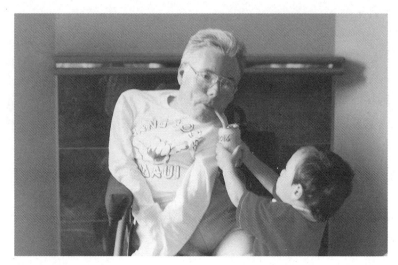

Always helpful, a young Jamie gives his Dad a drink. Janet Tkachyk

"He makes me take the dog for a walk. Then I have to make tea for him. Then he hollers, 'Clean your room.' He's so bossy," Keiko said with disgust.

"Do you sometimes wish you could go for a walk or play ball with him?"

"I've thought about it. But I don't mind him being in a wheelchair, 'cept when he starts ordering me around."

"Do you think your dad's pretty smart?"

"Maybe, but sometimes he acts so stupid. But he remembers a lot—millions of people's phone numbers."

"What's it like travelling on an airplane with your dad?"

"Tons of fun. He tells jokes to the stewardesses, and they all laugh."

"You know all about his frog-breathing?"

"Yeah. I made a Father's Day card for him, with a picture of a frog with its mouth open wide. The card said, 'Happy Frogger's Day'."

"You made it yourself?"

"Sure, I make all my cards."

Thus ended the animated conversation with Keiko. Apart from telling the author "Mon nom est Jamie"—something he had learned at his French immersion school—Jamie was disinclined to talk about anything apart from his new book of riddles and jokes.

. . . . .

SOMETIMES IT'S EASY TO FORGET that Gary is quite incapable of feeding himself a single morsel. In a restaurant or even at a banquet, his friends consider it just a matter of course to look after his needs in between their own bites. At one time Karen O'Neill, Gary's associate at the Canadian Wheelchair Sports Association (CWSA), got so involved in conversation that she found herself eating from Gary's plate and loading up his spoon from her own. "I guess it's because we all felt so integrated with him," she said. Jamie started feeding his dad when he was only two and a half. Louise Nkunzi, Gary's attendant at the time, remembers Jamie trying to manipulate stringy spaghetti into his dad's mouth with fair success. But when much of the sauce got smudged across Gary's face, Jamie solved the problem by licking it off himself.

As the ambulatory mother, Val carries the major responsibility for the day-to-day upbringing and nurturing of Keiko and Jamie. But she relies a lot on Gary, confident of his real interest in the kids' activities and in his gift of communication with people of all ages. "Sometimes they need someone to come in and talk to them. Thankfully they respond very well to Gary," Val said. Asked for her views about marriage, she answered, "You need trust, friendship and good emotional support. A sense of humour is helpful, and you've got to be flexible and not have too many rules."

Rodney, Gary's younger brother who as a ten-year-old pushed Gary's wheelchair to Getty's campaign office, can't speak too highly of Val. "Her level of dedication and commitment is phenomenal." Lee Sanderson, nurse and family friend, said, "It's amazing that Val was willing to take on the responsibility of a husband who'd been confined to an institution for so many years." When Gary's personal attendant is off or away, Val has to take over Gary's care and to put him to bed and look after him and his respirator during the night.

Louise Nkunzi worked as Gary's attendant for six years, reluctantly leaving a warm and loving home and a couple of very bright and active kids. She saw the hospitality too. When Randy Dickinson from New Brunswick was visiting Alberta, Gary invited him and a blind friend for dinner. They all arrived unannounced. Val was busy preparing dinner and looking after the kids, but she welcomed them in. Then two more guests and a dog showed up. "It took a little time," Randy said, "but she gave us an excellent meal and made us all feel at ease."

Asked about precious mementoes and treasures, Gary immediately spoke in glowing terms of two items in the bedroom that are placed "so I can see them first thing in the morning." One is a porcelain Mexican hat made by Keiko a couple of years ago and presented to her dad as a gift filled with caramel candies.

The other is a clapper or noise-maker that Jamie bought on his own for his dad just before Christmas. Afterwards, he told his mother, "When Dad goes anywhere, he can't clap his hands like everyone else. With this, he can." And it proved to be so—Gary can just grasp it in his left hand to make a slight clapping sound. The simple plastic clapper merited a fair-sized headline above an article by Cam Tait in the *Edmonton Journal*, entitled "How about a Round of Applause for a Son's Great Idea?"[1] The clapper may be made of cheap plastic, but Gary calls it one of the richest gifts he has ever received. He freely admits getting all choked up whenever he thinks of Jamie's unique gift.

22 | Governor General's Study Conference

THE YEAR WAS 1991. At the University of British Columbia in Vancouver, 225 people from across the nation had gathered for a three-day conference. Held every four to five years, that year's Governor General's Canadian Study Conference would focus on the theme "National Unity." Among the delegates, most ranging in age from twenty-five to forty, was a cheerful fellow in a wheelchair, Gary McPherson.

The *raison d'être* for the study conferences was a noble one: "to build unity and understanding among Canadians." The names of possible participants were put forward for consideration by the committee for that year. Every province and territory had representatives, chosen for their evident or potential leadership qualities, which included creativity, some experience in problem solving, good social skills, an appreciation of teamwork and the ability to handle adversity.

The 1991 participants included one First Nations man and one disabled person. The program chairperson was Rosalie Abella, an Ontario judge, and the chairman, John Cleghorn, president and CEO of the Royal Bank of Canada. Speakers for the three-day assembly included astronaut Marc Garneau, disabled athlete Rick Hansen and First Nations grand chief Ovid Mercredi.

After the three-day conference ended, the 225 participants were divided up into groups of fifteen and sent to areas throughout the country, where regional committees, made up of alumni from previous conferences, had prepared a ten-day "experience" for them. None of the fifteen knew where they were going nor who their companions would be. It was, in a sense, a venture into the unknown.

Gary's group toured through an area of central Quebec, visiting a huge hydroelectric plant, a pulp mill, a literacy program and a hockey stick manufacturer. Inspecting huge industrial plants was interesting, but just as interesting was learning about the literacy program and how people's lives are changed when they learn to read and write. Gary described it as "an eye-opening experience" from beginning to end.

They stayed in hotels and in private homes. The organizers had arranged for the group of fifteen to meet all kinds of people, including a "hard-core separatist," a farmwoman who met them at lunch one day. Despite her inability to speak any English, they parted as friends, with warm handshakes and hugs. Gary likes to think that she may have changed her attitude towards "English Canada," as former Quebec premier Lucien Bouchard called non-Quebecers.

For Gary, the most enriching experience was living and travelling with fourteen other people for the ten days in Quebec. They had left as strangers; they ended up as a team. His teammates lifted him and his wheelchair off and onto the school bus at least six times a day, and hauled him up steps into office buildings and hotels. Not only did they do all this willingly, but they soon grew to appreciate the importance of wheel-chair accessibility. At some places that were completely inaccessible to a wheelchair, they said, "If Gary can't go, we won't go in either."

Gary valued the companionship of Richard Powless, an aboriginal man from a reserve in Ontario. A soft-spoken person, he shared with the others the good and not-so-good things about life on the reserve. Another person who impressed Gary was Dianne Haskett, who later became mayor of London, Ontario. Dianne expressed her deep concern for the future of

Canada and left saying, "We must open up our homes and our hearts to those from other regions."

At the end of the ten days, the fifteen groups reconvened for a three-day plenary session at Laval University in Quebec City. Each group was asked to make a twenty-minute presentation, trying to capture the ten-day experience. They had plenty of freedom for creativity and ingenuity, interspersing straight reports with skits and songs. In attendance were the overall chairman, John Cleghorn, and Governor General Ray Hnatyshyn, both of whom asked questions and evaluated the presentations.

The first Study Conference had taken place in 1983. After participating in a conference, a delegate cannot return a second time but can help with forthcoming conferences as an alumnus. Participants are invited from various sectors: business, community, government and labour. Costs for the conference are met by contributions from business firms, labour organizations and the federal government. Gary believes it is money well spent. The hope is that each participant will return to his or her community as an enriched person with a better understanding of Canada, and an enhanced ability and desire to contribute to the community, workplace and family.

In 1995, Gary attended the Study Conference in Saskatoon, where he served as chair of the regional committee responsible for selecting Albertan participants and helping to create a program for the tour of the fifteen people heading to Alberta after the first session. Gary put forward the name of Walter Lawrence as someone who could be counted upon to make a valid contribution. Walter, a total quadriplegic, had a powerful effect on the able-bodied people who travelled with him and on those he met on tour. A modest, self-effacing sort of fellow, Walter would only go so far as to say, "The effect I had on others might have been significant only because of the common misconceptions around disabilities."

In April 1999, at the Ottawa residence of the Governor General, Gary attended the board meeting for the organizing committee of the upcoming 2000 Study Conference. They chose the beautiful Banff Centre as the venue with Eric Newell, CEO of Syncrude Canada, as general chairman and the secretariat in Edmonton. "Gary's the reason I'm doing this job," Eric said later. "He's so persuasive."

The two had met five years previously when Eric and Premier Ralph Klein co-chaired the Alberta Economic Development Authority, an organization set up to study economic strategies for the province. As chairman of the Premier's Council at the time, Gary wrote a letter stating that they should have a representative from the disabled community. He later received a reply turning down his request. But persistent fellow that he is, Gary refused to be deterred and later phoned Eric, asking if they might meet for breakfast "to discuss things."

It turned out that they shared mutual interests in Canada's social development—which they rated to be just as important as its economic development—and in the welfare of disabled and socially marginalized people. In a short time they became good friends: the affable, high-profile CEO with a host of volunteer commitments and the wheelchair-wielding crusader for the disabled, with a head brimful of ideas. Eric got even with Gary by asking him to sit on the executive of the committee for the 2000 Study Group to serve as vice-chair of community resources.

The theme for the Study Group's meeting in Banff was "Strengthening the Community and Developing Tomorrow's Leaders." As with previous conferences, the 225 participants at the three-day conference found themselves taking notes furiously in order to retain as much as they could of the lectures and presentations. Then they dispersed in groups of fifteen, to meet again ten days later on May 31 at Laval University in Quebec City in the presence of Governor General Adrienne Clarkson.

While at Banff, Eric Newell and Gary McPherson shared their views about Canadian society. Both are aware of the importance of economic growth or stability, but both deplore any growth that excludes social concerns. Both want our society to be inclusive; no one should be left out. Gary wants the disabled and socially disadvantaged to be enabled, not pampered or coddled.

Eric insists that business leaders have a responsibility to their communities. "They simply cannot be locked up in the walls of their company." Same with university leaders: they cannot work away in academic isolation as if the community around them did not exist. Gary, working from the volunteer side, believes that the private sector, labour and government need to work at problems together. Community-based solutions are far more likely to be effective than those handed down from Ottawa.

As general chair of the 2000 conference, Eric Newell championed the study conferences as a great boon for Canada. He was highly appreciative of the work of Gary McPherson in three consecutive conferences. "He's an example of the leadership capacity that we build in people who take part. We'll see the benefits of this Banff conference ten years from now when these people are running all kinds of enterprises and learning to handle the issues and concerns of the day."

23 | Gary McPherson, Author

*People seldom tap into their deepest strengths and abilities until forced
to do so by a major adversity....The terrible experiences of our lives,
despite the pain they bring, may become our redemption....You can
acquire a learning/coping response as an alternative to feeling like a
victim that blames others.*

—DR. AL SIEBERT, author of *The Survivor Personality*[1]

GARY NEVER COMPLETED HIGH SCHOOL. During his youthful
years on Stations 32 and 67 in the University Hospital, he much preferred
the study of math and science to literature and English. As a member of
the Jaycees, he learned the basics of public speaking and report writing.
During his years of holding executive and administrative jobs with
wheelchair sports and advocacy groups for the disabled, he learned how
to analyze and study abstract ideas and concepts, an ability that received
fine-tuning during his chairmanship of the Premier's Council.

But none of that inspired him to write. One day, however, he realized
he had a message to tell. For one thing, he felt that his life experience
was unique—struck by a disabling disease that took the lives of a host of

sufferers, he had survived and in the process learned much about survival. Institutionalized for thirty-four years of his life, he acquired in-depth knowledge about health services and medical care as an astute observer on the receiving end.

And so he began to write. His works of varying lengths included a learned paper bearing the curious title "A Monkey Shakes the Tree," used to address the National Rehabilitation Conference in Halifax in October 1995. Among other things, Gary spoke about the importance of motivating factors and the relationship to success in the rehabilitation of disabled people.[2]

In 2000 he published *With Every Breath I Take: One Person's Extraordinary Journey to a Healthy Life, and How You Can Share in It,* a nontechnical book written for the general reader which presents, in essence, Gary's personal philosophy as it relates to a healthy lifestyle. In no way does he lament the illness that confined him to a lifetime in a wheelchair. Rather, he begins with the words of the legendary blind and deaf Helen Keller: "I thank God for my handicaps, for through them, I have found myself, my work and my God." Gary states that he wouldn't trade his experiences, friendships, relationships and life for anything.

The book begins with his life on the polio ward "when I was too busy fighting for the next breath of air and surviving from one medical crisis to the next." A few years later, when the crisis era had passed, he responded to a questionnaire, which asked, among other questions, "Are you in good health?" He simply refused to say no: he was disabled but not unhealthy.

Gary advocates focusing less on disease and illness, and more on good health and whoever and whatever promotes it. "If we want people to take responsibility for their health, we must give them the tools. This means changing the culture and our whole approach to personal health."

He believes that "virtually everything we do and everything around us can affect our health in some way."[3] His book presents what he has found to be beneficial to physical, emotional and spiritual health, summarized under easy-to-remember acronyms. For better physical health, he advises, follow the WISER approach, which may be loosely summerized as:

W – water is essential for good health; drink lots of it.

I – inhale deeply several times a day.

S – slow down when eating and chew your food well.

E – exercise your body and your mind.

R – rest and sleep enough for your body's needs.[4]

Gary aims to guzzle down eight glasses of water a day. His advice is to do deep breathing exercises several times a day, something he has never been able to do. Good dietary habits include steering clear of fatty and starchy foods. He quotes Dr. Spock, who recommends reducing intake of meat and dairy products, provided that the intake of vegetables, fruits and whole grains is abundant. Gary believes that people battling a weight problem wouldn't feel the need to eat so much if their meals consisted of nutritious food.

Exercising every day (or at least three times a week) is essential to good health. It's not easy for him, but he rides an exercise bike, having just enough strength in his left leg to get the pedals on both sides turning. The amount of sleep required varies from person to person, but a persistent sleep deficit can be detrimental to good health, having especially harmful effects on the immune system.

For emotional, psychological and spiritual health, he promotes FAITH:

F – forgiveness of yourself and others.

A – acceptance of people and situations.

I – integrity in all aspects of our lives.

T – trust in our fellow man and ourselves.

H – honesty, humility and humour.[5]

"If you don't have faith it is very difficult if not impossible to be effective, let alone be happy and healthy."[6] To Gary, faith means trust and hope in yourself, in God, and your family and friends. "Studies show that people who have a strong faith are healthier and live longer than those who don't." Thoughts are important too—always try to feed your mind with constructive thoughts.

In the belief that "intangibles" affect our physical, emotional and spiritual health, Gary advises continually nourishing emotional and spiritual needs. Volunteer, help out and give to other people. You need hope: without it, people just drift through life like a ship with no one at the helm. A person blessed with a good sense of humour will find the road of life less rocky. Fear of failure is common to everyone and sucks all the joy from life. As the Bible says, love can cast out fear.

Gary places high emphasis on a person's spiritual needs, and he believes in the power of meditation to combat stress and the power of prayer to enhance health. "Prayer seems to be particularly effective when it is complemented with words of love and praise."[7]

He quotes the Russian author Alexander Solzhenitsyn: "Let us admit, even if in a whisper and only to ourselves: in this bustle of life at breakneck speed—what are we living for?" Insofar as his own health is concerned, Gary is about as pragmatic as one can get: "I want the energy and stamina to do what I want, when I want, and with whomever I want."[8]

Gary concludes his book with a strong plea for people to change the way they look at health. He believes that we must design a health care system which promotes health and wellness, and minimizes—but does not neglect—disease and illness. Each person must strive towards a healthier lifestyle. Government health care programs will not do that for us: each of us must make that responsibility our own. The old axiom consisting of ten two-letter words says it all: "If it is to be, it is up to me."

Gary's book might never be a best-seller, but certainly it will make a difference in the lives of its readers.

24 | Stronger by Weakness

Peter Singer, professor of bioethics at Princeton University, has written a controversial book called Practical Ethics. *In his book Singer suggests, amongst other things, that killing a cat is a more serious moral ill than killing a child with a disability.*

—DAVID HINGSBURGER[1]

MANY PEOPLE LISTENING to CBC-Radio on May 23, 2001, were appalled, even nauseated, that anyone could make such a claim. Had our society sunk so low? How could anyone schooled in human ethics have such a dismal regard for human life?

Gary McPherson heard the "Ideas" radio program that broadcast Singer's claim. Inwardly he might have seethed, but outwardly his reaction was muted. He had run into lots of "Singers" in his lifetime—people who saw little use or place in our society for the disabled. But he would not allow such a statement to go unchallenged. In a March 2003 article for the *Archives of Physical and Rehabilitation Medicine*, he and Professor Dick Sobsey rebutted Singer's inflammatory statement in no uncertain terms.

Still, Gary could not deny that many questions had been asked. What is the purpose of keeping people alive who will never get better? Why devote resources and costly care on people who apparently have nothing to contribute to society? Why perpetuate the lives of those—the feeble-minded, the blind and incurably crippled—whose quality of life is deemed to be abysmally low?

Why not "purify our race" as the eugenicists once argued by getting rid of people with stunted minds or deformed and decaying bodies? By careful use of good, selective stock, we could make our human species genetically pure, healthy, strong and productive. A good cattle breeder could show us the way.

"We need to discuss 'Do not resuscitate' with you." With these words the doctor on intensive care confronted Anita Dadson and her husband. Their thirty-one-year-old daughter with cerebral palsy had been admitted with breathing problems and needed to be put on a respirator. The parents were aghast. There was no doubt what the doctor had in mind: no special effort would be made to save her life.[2]

Dr. Gregor Wolbring, born a "Thalidomide baby" with no legs, teaches biochemistry and bioethics at the University of Calgary. "Nothing really surprises me anymore regarding the devaluation of disabled people's lives," he said. "We have this dismal record about disabled people, because we view them as really not worth living, and they're really better off dead or not being born."

In his book *Our Own Master Race*, Dr. Angus McLaren of the University of Victoria says that the sentiments involved in dehumanizing people with disabilities is nothing new. "The tolerant society we believe Canada to be is more mythical than real when it comes to disability," he wrote. David Hingsburger, a writer and therapist who works with the developmentally disabled, believes that people with disabilities "have managed to transcend societal messages that we all must live in perfect bodies with perfect hair."

Why do we have this attitude, not only of intolerance but of fear and embarrassment in the presence of disabled people? Gary McPherson first encountered it when a barmaid refused to serve him. Some years later, a waitress in a restaurant turned to Val and asked what Gary would like to order. "Why don't you just ask him?" said Val.

Walter Lawrence, a total quadriplegic, recalls his attitude during his pre-injury days. "I remember this young woman in a wheelchair, hurrying because she was late for her class. I desperately wanted to give her a hand," he said, "but I'd run by as if I didn't see her." Gary's sister Kim Worth gets really heated up when she hears someone say that if they were disabled by a serious accident or crippling disease, they would rather die. "I feel almost like hitting such a person," she fumed, "because I know people like Gary who are living life to the full."

In its status report for the 1998–99 fiscal year, the Alberta Human Rights and Citizenship Commission reported that complaints filed on the basis of discrimination over physical and mental disability dominated all other types of complaints during the year.[3] Gary McPherson regrets seeing people "segmented by medical diagnosis," like a form of apartheid. He believes that once we start putting labels on people, we denigrate them.

Brent Foster, coach of the Canadian Men's Wheelchair Basketball Team at the 1992 Barcelona Olympics, freely admitted the weird attitude he once had towards disabled people. "I had this stereotype, I just felt uncomfortable around them, didn't know what to say or how to act." After his contact with the basketball players of the Alberta Northern Lights, he realized that "the problem was in my mind, an image problem." He was taken aback when he first met Gary, but later he said, "There is no man that I respect more or am more proud of than Gary. He is the epitome of manliness."·

Disabled athletes can be classified according to the degree of their handicap. Although Gary is obviously not an athlete, he would be ranked in Class 1A, the most disabled. Someone has called him, paradoxically, one of the most disabled and least disabled people. And according to Ernie Daigle, Gary's barber for forty years, "he wants disabled people to have their rightful place in our society." He wants them to be proactive, to take control of their lives and to get out of the often-imposed state of learned helplessness. Confined to a wheelchair for forty-six years, Eric Boyd firmly believes in "honing the residual skills that you have. That's the way to make meaning out of your life and its circumstances."

Self-image and confidence is, of course, important to everyone, not just those with disabilities. A person's attitude or outlook can turn things around completely. Dr. Jim Vargo suffered a broken neck and quadriplegia when he was twelve, yet he went on to become a professor in the Faculty of Rehabilitation Medicine at the University of Alberta. One of the most popular professors before he retired, Jim believed that "if you can't change your fate, change your attitude." He said, chuckling: "I'm ninety percent dependent insofar as self-care goes, but I'm ninety percent independent in leisure and productivity."

Do the disabled have much to give? Jim Allen believes they have the gift of friendship. "When you have friends who are handicapped, the friendship is rarely one-sided. The benefits to someone like myself in knowing Clayton and Gary were great beyond measure."

Some seriously disabled people have made outstanding contributions. One of the most incapacitated people on the face of the earth is Stephen Hawking, afflicted for many years with amyotrophic lateral sclerosis (ALS, or Lou Gehrig's disease). He has no speech and no bodily movement except for a slight pincers action between one thumb and index finger. Gary had lunch with Hawking, probably the world's foremost astrophysicist, one day and learned firsthand that the disability does not interfere with his ability to think and theorize. Alfred Nobel, the creator of dynamite and the man for whom the Nobel Prize is awarded, was so severely disabled physically as a child that for a long time he was kept out of school. Beaver, Gary's roommate for many years on the polio ward, learned computer programming, becoming so skilled that a firm hired him for full-time work.

Since the early 1990s, the Robert Latimer case has served to rally and unite the voices of the disabled community like no other highly publicized event. After appealing all the way up to the Supreme Court of

Canada, in 2001 Latimer's sentence was upheld: life imprisonment with no parole for ten years for the killing of his daughter Tracy, afflicted with cerebral palsy and said to be in pain all the time. Many Canadians felt strongly that the sentence was far too severe for what was clearly a "mercy killing."

But several groups representing families and people with disabilities were outraged at any suggestion of leniency. Some said there is no ethical argument for killing people with disabilities. Latimer claimed he was acting compassionately to relieve his daughter of terrible pain. But Gary questioned "How do we know this was a crime of compassion? Mr. Latimer could have committed his crime out of hate."[4]

Dr. Dick Sobsey, professor in the developmental disabilities program at the University of Alberta and a leading expert on the abuse of people with disabilities, analyzed the Latimer case and others like it, with the conclusion that "the crimes are simply not important because the victim is not important." Lucy Gwin, the flamboyant editor of *Mouth*, a disability rights magazine, had strong words about the Latimer case: "As long as we publicly devalue the lives of people with disabilities...then Tracy Latimer is going to die."

If the Latimer case has helped to bring disabled people "out of the closet," all well and good. Now is a good time, according to Gary McPherson, for them to set goals for themselves and establish their needs. Since most of them have ailments that can't be "fixed," maximum efforts should be made to improve their quality of life. Rehabilitation must focus on optimizing existing strengths and abilities. And, as Gary has frequently stated, individuals with disabilities need to be proactive, setting their own lifestyles and taking responsibility for their own health. "We don't have as much room for error in terms of how we conduct our lives," Gary said. "We just don't have strong, vigorous bodies and therefore have to take special care of them."

Gary has never felt comfortable with either charity or pity. He's glad that his fellow members in the Jaycees never gave him any breaks. As an advocate for people with disabilities, his goal is for them to be given a chance to live useful and fulfilling lives, and, if possible, to be steady and productive workers. But he worries about the state of affairs in Alberta, and says that with the prosperity ethos riding high on the agenda and the "let's get everyone working" objective, opportunities to start small businesses, get job training and attain education abound. Unfortunately, many disabled people don't qualify. Gary worries even more that the voice of the disability community will not be heard unless there are qualified spokespersons and advocates looking after their interests. Regrettably, "we are not growing many new advocates, and the only way change happens is through intelligent and persistent advocacy."

It's hard not to be impressed with the opinion of people who are intimate friends or who have worked closely with Gary McPherson. Bob Chelmick, formerly an Edmonton television announcer and now a radio producer, spent hours recording interviews with Gary on videotape. He believes Gary has aimed high. "He has striven to make the best of what he has, to understand himself and how he fits within the universe and creation." Randy Dickinson, executive-director of the New Brunswick Premier's Council on the Status of Disabled Persons, remains firmly convinced that Gary's influence for the good of people with disabilities has stretched far beyond the province of Alberta.

25 | Disabled Heroes

I've seen so many people with a disability who overcame adversity and went on to make amazing contributions...they are the real heroes.

—DR. BOB STEADWARD,
Founder and President of the International Paralympic Committee and Director of the Steadward Centre, University of Alberta[1]

SOME ARE WELL KNOWN and often in the public eye; others live quiet lives in obscurity. Some are blind, some mentally challenged, some are coping with cerebral palsy, some with Lou Gehrig's disease, some with the aftermath of polio, some with brain or spinal injuries. A few have found the onslaught of such devastating disease or injury overwhelming, and they have succumbed physically or emotionally. But most have carried on, spurred by what might be called the indomitable human spirit. The majority lead quality lives, thankful to be alive and rarely giving much thought to their disability. The presence of a quiet, inner strength in their person is nearly always unmistakable. Many of these disabled heroes contribute to the needs of other people; their contributions to a myriad of worthy causes and enterprises are, according to Bob Steadward, "amazing."

The names of some of these disabled heroes are firmly fixed in history. Helen Keller, left blind and deaf as an infant after an attack of meningitis, went on to write books and give lectures and be interviewed by heads of state. As Gary McPherson wrote in the introduction to his book, she was actually able to thank God for her multiple disabilities. Stephen Hawking is venerated throughout the world for his wisdom and innovative thinking in the fields of cosmology and astrophysics. His book *A Brief History of Time* remains a best-seller.

Terry Fox and Rick Hansen played wheelchair basketball together on the same championship team, the Vancouver Cable Cars. Terry became a national hero when he walked halfway across Canada on an artificial leg. Terry Fox Runs, held continually over the years since he died, have raised millions of dollars for cancer research. Rick Hansen's monumental Man in Motion world tour made him a legendary figure. His work on behalf of people with spinal injuries and the cause of the disabled goes on, radiating out from the Rick Hansen Institute at the University of British Columbia. Without Rick's efforts and determination, it is doubtful if the Alberta Premier's Council for the Status of Persons with Disabilities would have seen the light of day.

People with memories of World War II will tell you about Sir Douglas Bader, the famous British fighter pilot who lost both his legs but refused to stop flying. At Gary's request, in August 1977 Bader attended the Canadian Games for the Physically Disabled in Edmonton as guest of honour, officially opening the games. Gary's friend Jim Allen, who escorted sixty-five-year-old Bader and his wife on a sightseeing tour of Edmonton, called him "a remarkable human being with great drive and tenacity." Bader received a knighthood from the Queen, not for his heroic flying record during the war but for his work with disabled people.

There are, of course, plenty of disabled heroes right in our backyard. The extraordinary and lovable Cam Tait hasn't let cerebral palsy interfere with his writing a regular column, "Our Community," for the *Edmonton Journal* since 1979. A first meeting with Cam may make the listener strain a little to get the gist of his laboured speech, but you quickly become

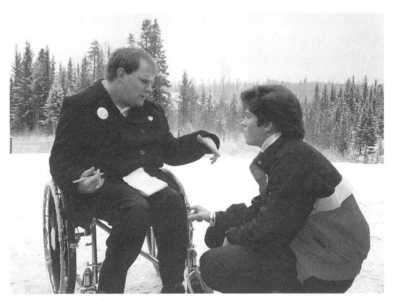

Cam Tait interviews Amanda Hansen as her husband, Rick, completes the Man in Motion World Tour in 1987. Janet Tkachyk

aware of the man's gentle wit and wisdom. Cam has achieved a fine reputation as a humorist and raconteur and has made public presentations to many groups, including the staff of Imperial Oil and Grant MacEwan Community College. As Gary has testified, "Everyone in Edmonton knows and loves Cam Tait."

Connie Clarke (now Packer) was hit with polio in 1953 and lived for twelve years on Stations 32 and 67, near Gary and "the boys." Like Gary, her breathing is severely impaired, requiring her to use a pneumobelt around her waist, and she has no movement except in her right hand. Yet Connie is one of the most optimistic people you could possibly meet and the possessor of a strong, living faith in God. With a paintbrush or a pencil taped or strapped to her finger, she paints landscapes and writes poems. Connie is the archivist for the family of former polio patients and their families, and the focal point for the occasional reunions.

At age twelve, Jim Vargo fell from a tree and broke his neck. He was confined to a wheelchair but managed to complete high school, then went on to the University of Alberta, where he eventually got his B.A. and later, a Ph.D. in counselling psychology. He would not have had the courage to tackle university had a couple of health professionals not laid the cards on the table for him. "Jim," they said, "you're paralyzed from the neck down but not from the neck up." That gave him the confidence he needed. He went on to become an associate dean in the Faculty of Rehabilitation Medicine, and in 1994 he was named Canadian Professor of the Year. The overwhelming choice among forty-one nominees for the award, Jim was described in the citation as "a role model not only because of his invigorating teaching methods, but also because of the inspirational example he sets every day for his students, colleagues, and the university community." Jim's list, "Ten Things I've Learned about Teaching," published in an alumni magazine, has become a classic.[2]

At birth the nerves to both his arms were stretched during a difficult breech delivery, and Bill Watson was born with paralyzed arms. But by the age of three he had learned to play with toys and to feed himself with his feet. With iron grit and skillful manipulation, young Billy Watson trained those feet to become substitute hands, hands that would get him through school and later to the University of Alberta. In 1928 he graduated with a law degree. William Watson Lodge in Kananaskis Country, west of Calgary, is a wonderful facility specially designed for people in wheelchairs but available for a variety of disability groups.

The August 2001 issue of *Status Report*, published by the Premier's Council on the Status of Persons with Disabilities, reported the feats of two blind mountain climbers. Ross Watson of Cochrane, Alberta, was the first blind person to scale Canada's highest peak, Mount Logan in the Yukon, which towers to 6,050 metres (19,850 feet). On May 25, 2001, Erik Weihenmayer of Englewood, Colorado, reached the summit of Mount Everest, at 8,848 metres (29,029 feet), the world's highest mountain. Suffering complete loss of vision at the age of thirteen from glaucoma, Weihenmayer hasn't allowed blindness to keep him from becoming a popular speaker and writer, nor to interfere with his enjoyment of scuba diving, marathon running and skiing.[3]

Audrie Fletcher was born with spina bifida, which left her with flail, floppy legs. As a child she got around fairly well with braces and elbow crutches, and she was a good student at school. In her adolescent years she underwent several orthopedic operations to stabilize her floppy legs, but unfortunately, they failed. Audrie had to use a wheelchair for the rest of her life. Then, as so often happens, other congenital abnormalities insidiously took over and ruined what little good health she had. She spent her latter years in constant pain. After all these setbacks, did she do much with her life? Some people might say no, well, nothing really noteworthy. Perhaps, but most of her friends and family members would likely answer that Audrie excelled in making cheerful phone calls and sending encouraging notes far and wide. Before she died in Calgary in 1975, her relatively cheerless life had brightened the lives of countless others.

Walter Lawrence was only seventeen when his head hit a hard object after a dive into Okanagan Lake, near Kelowna, British Columbia. The impact damaged his spinal cord high up in the neck, causing instant paralysis; he floated helplessly until his friends rescued him from drowning. Walter lost all feeling below his neck and, like Gary, his diaphragm was paralyzed, necessitating a tracheotomy and the use of a ventilator twenty-four hours a day. He stayed in Pearson Hospital, in Vancouver, for fifteen years, until he finally mastered some head and neck manoeuvres that got air into and out of his lungs. He still uses a ventilator at night.

Far from a life of inactivity, Walter works as a peer counsellor and mentor at the G.F. Strong Rehab Centre in Vancouver, a facility for the rehabilitation of brain- and spinal-injured persons. He counsels the families and the injured people, most of whom are far less disabled than he. He "propels" his wheelchair by turning his head and blowing into or sucking on little tubes that in some mysterious fashion control the mechanism of his wheelchair.

"I believe we human beings need opportunities to give and to contribute," Walter said. "This is contrary to popular belief that we should be trying to get all we can for ourselves. That idea is all wrong." As refreshing a person as anyone could meet, he knows all kinds of wrapped-up-in-themselves people with no physical disability whatsoever, but for whom life is almost unbearable.

For Walter and his wife Wendy, the jewel in their lives is their four-year-old adopted daughter Geneva, who came from an orphanage in China. Walter thanks his friend Gary McPherson for this precious gift. Gary had a friend in Ontario who adopted a Chinese baby, and he suggested that Walter contact this person. It took time, but eventually Walter and Wendy got their reward. "She's an absolute gem," he said, "and has blessed us and given us so much."

Both Walter Lawrence and Gary McPherson are about as disabled as it is possible to be. Yet they live abundant lives, thankful for each day and well aware that their hold on life has at times been precarious and remains far from secure. Both are spiritual, and both pray. Walter says of Gary, "He wants to give away to enhance the lives of other people. He wants to see everyone benefit from whatever he can contribute. He'll go the extra mile for you."

26 | Awards and Friendships

OVER THE COURSE OF TWENTY-NINE YEARS, Gary has received tributes, accolades and honours in recognition of his work and contributions in a variety of areas of endeavour. Twenty-eight plaques, awards and scrolls have come his way, enough to cover the four walls of a trophy room.

But if you go looking for a trophy room, or even just a trophy wall, in Gary and Val's modest home in Edmonton's Riverbend district, you'll look in vain. True, you will find above his computer a clock with a plaque displaying his 1994 Award of Merit from the Edmonton Sports Reporters' Association. On an adjacent wall hangs the certificate for his honorary doctorate and the picture taken at his retirement from the Canadian Wheelchair Sports Association. But there are no awards to be seen anywhere else.

If you speak nicely to Val, she will escort you downstairs to an ordinary unfinished basement room, where you will find three large, unpadded cardboard boxes overflowing with framed awards and laurels and engraved plaques. But be prepared to dust them off if you want to read them. None of them ordinarily see the light of day.

About the only way you can get Gary to talk about all these marvellous ego-enhancing tributes is to ask if there are any he considers

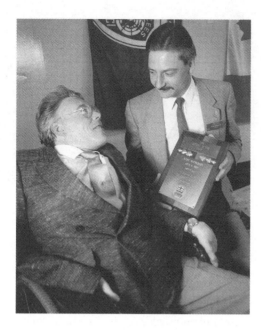

especially meaningful. And there are some. The first decoration he was given, the Rookie of the Year Award by the Jaycees in 1969, meant a lot to him. More than thirty years later, it still retains special significance. In an organization of able-bodied individuals he was singled out, not because he was disabled but because of what he had done in and for the organization. Further, it was a special honour for him to be included on the list with previous winners, all of whom he considered "pretty impressive." When the Jaycees put forward his name for Citizen of the Year in 1987, he was really surprised. He had left the organization in 1971 and thought everyone would have forgotten all about him.

Being inducted into the Sports Hall of Fame is a bright feather in anyone's cap. In 1991 Gary was honoured by the Edmonton Sports Hall of Fame for "ten years in the interest of sports in general, especially that of basketball." Two years later he was nominated to the Alberta Sports Hall of Fame for "outstanding contribution to the sport of wheelchair basketball." He can't recall much about the latter event, saying that "Val would remember much more than I can." But he does recall that the ceremony

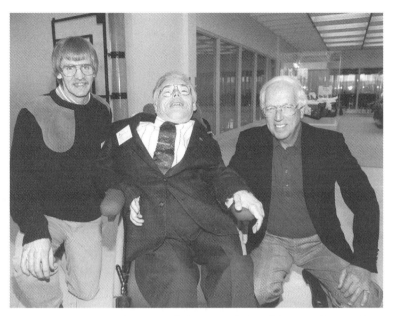

Wayne Bowes, Gary McPherson and Al McCann, left to right, were honored by the Alberta Sports Hall of Fame on May 28, 1993. Edmonton Journal

was held at the Capri Hotel in Red Deer and that other inductees included Mark Tewksbury (swimming), Lanny McDonald (hockey) and John Helton (football). These awards are obviously dear to Gary's heart because they acknowledged him as one of the rare builders of sports for the disabled, in the same league as his good friend Bob Steadward.

The Integration Award bears an uninspiring name and consists of a plaque that forms the base for two interlocking circles of copper alloy. But it means much to Gary. It was presented to him in 1997 by the Alberta Association of Community Living, one of whose goals is the integration of mentally disabled people, including those with Down's syndrome, into the community. Gary said that when he was with the Premier's Council on the Status of Persons with Disabilities, the emphasis was on the physical side of disabilities, an area that he knew "like the back of my hand." He knew he would have to work hard to understand the issues and challenges around people with developmental (mental) disabilities, and he did just that. It was particularly gratifying to be acknowledged for the contribution he had made towards facilitating the work of groups supporting the cause of the mentally disabled.

When you mention the 1994 Robert Jackson Award for outstanding contributions to the Canadian Wheelchair Sports Association, Gary smiles with satisfaction. It was special, he said, not for the honour conferred upon him but because of "the outstanding people I worked with in basketball, people who were not only colleagues but also became close friends." They included Dr. Robert Jackson, orthopedic surgeon with the Toronto Argonauts, who pioneered wheelchair sports in Canada and who was also the first doctor to operate on the knees of Bobby Orr, the Boston Bruins' great defenceman.

Among the dust-covered trophies in Gary's basement is one that he doesn't hesitate to include with the more official ones, a framed "Backseat Driver's Licence." It was presented to him in 1978 by Reenie Kinch, a lady friend of bygone years who obviously understood his idiosyncrasies. He admits to having been accused over the years of directing traffic from the sidelines or the backseat. Val thinks he is pretty good at backseat vacuuming and housecleaning. Now that he has a licence, he can say that he is legitimate.

From his base at the Aberhart Hospital, Gary coached a mixed slow-pitch ball team for seventeen years. He's not sure when the players got together to present him with a "Coaching Award by the Bad News AIRS Team for Outstanding Support and Coaching." He reckons alumni for the team number well over one hundred, nearly all of whom were "great people."

Another honour that took him completely by surprise was the 1978 Award for Outstanding Contribution to the Disabled in Canada, presented by the Canadian Rehabilitation Council for the Disabled. Gary and his parents had travelled to Calgary for the ceremony at the Four Seasons hotel. The award honours a person who has acted as an advocate to better the lot of disabled people in general. Gary's efforts up until that time had been directed to sports for the disabled, and he was surprised to receive the award because at that time the beneficial value of sports in enhancing the quality of life of people with disabilities was not generally recognized. In time, sport would be seen as having "more of an impact on the lives of disabled people than many would admit," Gary said.

After serving for ten years as chairman of the Premier's Council, in 1998 Gary received a certificate "in recognition of contribution to the enhancement and promotion of full and equal participation by people with disabilities." He appreciated the recognition for his long period of service in a demanding, high-profile job, but says he "didn't need the accolades."

One of the laurels that caused Gary to chuckle to himself hangs on the wall above his computer: the 1994 Edmonton Sports Reporters' Association Award of Merit. Back in 1978, in the early days of the Northern Lights, he had tried in vain to get any reporters interested in wheelchair basketball—with one exception: Cam Tait of the *Edmonton Journal*. George Ward of the *Journal's* sports department assigned Cam to travel with the Northern Lights on their road trips and cover the games for the newspaper. The young cub reporter got the chance to build his career as a writer, while giving the Northern Lights the media exposure they had been struggling to get. Fifteen years later Gary was asked to be a member of the committee that brought the 1994 Gold Cup world championship of wheelchair basketball to Edmonton. Gary still wonders why he was nominated for the Sports Reporters' Award—he thinks it was because of his involvement with the more recent Gold Cup tournament. It seemed ironic to be getting such recognition for relatively little effort, after being spurned by the press for so long.

· · · · ·

THE TROPHIES, plaques and scrolls that languish in boxes in a dingy basement room obviously don't rate all that high a priority in the McPherson cosmology. But in five minutes a casual visitor finds out what is important in the lives of Gary and Val—first their family, then their friends. The latter are legion.

But it could have been otherwise; Gary might well be spending his years in a friendless state. True, he had close buddies during those years on the polio ward, so close that they were more like brothers than friends. But with the exception of Beaver, they all have died. He certainly wasn't making friends with many of the nurses, who looked upon him as a "lippy" and "sassy" pest or brat. His sister Kim volunteered that sometimes he was "pretty mouthy." To nursing and hospital administration, he was a constant thorn in the flesh, always trying to break or bend hospital rules and recruiting others to join in the revolt.

Few would deny that he used sweet-talk or pressure to get people to do things for him. At one period, Gary was so preoccupied with himself that the needs and concerns of other people rarely penetrated his hard shell. Some people have described him as being too persuasive in his arguments and too tenacious in recruiting people for his various projects. For instance, he butted heads with a wheelchair basketball coach who was every bit as bull-headed as he was. Later, in a position of authority, he was accused of laziness and abusiveness of power. One person intimated that if Gary had escaped the polio epidemic, he would almost certainly have ended up in jail.

There may be some truth in all those statements—Gary did have feet of clay—but he learned, and he changed. He gained social graces and underwent a change of heart. "At one time he was pretty caustic in his comments and seemed to delight in rocking the boat," one long-term friend said. "But he has changed a lot, becoming much more kindly and polished."

An adage states that to have a friend, you must first be one. And Gary has been a friend, displaying caring, warmth, affection and regard for others—all qualities that make for genuine friendship. He has friends all across Canada and friends from all levels of society, something that doesn't surprise Vance Milligan. "His network of friends is unbelievably extensive," said Vance. One of his closest friends was Marshall Smith, who developed paraplegia following a rugby injury and subsequent unsuccessful surgery. Marshall knew Gary since 1981 when he became president of the BC division of the Canadian Wheelchair Basketball Association, during the time when Gary was head of the national group. They were friends ever since, often meeting at Marshall's place at Whistler, British Columbia. He said of Gary, "He's such a good friend and a thoughtful person with a great mind."[1]

Gary's mother, Dorothy, believes that Gary's capacity to connect with other people goes back a long way, even to his adolescent years on Station 67. Her husband, Roderick, tired, anxious and frustrated at the end of the day, would go up to visit Gary and come away feeling better about himself and the world.

In 1977, Carl Shields came to Edmonton from Laurentian University in Ontario to work with Gary as an administrative assistant with the Canadian Games for the Physically Disabled. Carl was much impressed with the determined efforts made by Gary to find him a place to live. He helped with the games and later assisted Gary with other projects, not as a subordinate, he maintains, but as a friend.

Gerry Way first met Gary in 1968 when the polio patients provided the important communication channels using their amateur radio setup on the ward. Over many years they worked together in wheelchair sports. "I still would rate him number one," Gerry said, thirty-one years later. "I would trust him for anything. And he's a delight to travel with."

Dr. Ted Aaron, one of the physicians caring for polio patients, remembers Gary and Clayton from those long-ago iron-lung days and has followed his career over the years. "He reached the stage of liking people and trying to bring out the best in them, rather than irritating them," he said. Recently he and Gary were together at the University of Alberta Faculty Club. He started to introduce Gary to several of his acquaintances, but most of them said, "Oh, we know Gary." Charlie Gardner, board member of the Northern Lights, has had a similar experience. "I can remember many times when I was pushing Gary in the wheelchair down the street and being constantly stopped by people who recognized him. Some of them were nice-looking girls too," he said. "As far as I'm concerned, Gary has been a friend all along."

Peter Eriksson, former coach of wheelchair basketball athletes in Sweden, said, "I'd would be happy to go out of my way to do anything for Gary at any time." Don Getty calls him "a strong, loyal friend."

Karen O'Neill, an associate of Gary's in the Canadian Wheelchair Basketball Association, has some understanding of Gary's capacity for friendship. "He never loses sight of all the things that matter to his friends. He has always had an appreciation of the accomplishments of people he knows. As a result, I think that many of us would be willing to do just about anything he asked of us."

Two people who feel exceedingly grateful to Gary are Randy Wyness and Ron Minor, both paraplegics who starred with the Alberta Northern Lights Wheelchair Basketball Team. His brother Rod also feels a debt of gratitude to Gary for helping him to gain confidence in social situations. "He taught me to sit down beside a stranger, introduce myself and not be afraid."

One day Fran Vargo and Gary, both of whom were representing the Premier's Council, had arrived in Calgary and were travelling to a meeting in a taxi. The taxi driver, a young woman called Linda, was soon telling them her life story and about her interest in the Sweet Adelines singing group. She asked if they would like to hear a new song she was learning, and they said yes. So they drove through the streets of Calgary, the young woman singing a short but beautiful melody to two people who were complete strangers.

Val and Gary both state that their love for Hawaii was not the only reason for choosing that location for their wedding. Both wanted a small wedding, but had they stayed in Canada, they would have had a real dilemma on their hands. "There's no way we could have invited all our friends," Val said, "and it would really have bothered us to leave anyone out. Gary has such a tremendous circle of friends."

Lack of mobility restricts Gary's freedom to maintain his network of friends; sometimes the telephone is his only means of keeping in touch. Gary's friend Chukwuemeka Obiajunwa, known as Meka, works in financial planning and has a small import-export business. Hailing from Nigeria, he has lived in Edmonton for many years, but he still does not feel ties strong enough to call it home. But there is one exception—his friendship with Gary. Meka confesses that Gary is the only person he can talk to freely, and they talk on the phone almost every day. "He's the only true friend I have. If I'm sad when I talk to him, I feel better afterwards. I believe that Gary may be severely disabled in order that he might become a channel of God's grace."

If long-standing friendships are any indication of a person's measure, then Gary can hold his head high. Judge Don Buchanan first met Gary and "the boys" in 1957, long before he entered law school. They have never lost contact, even if the get-togethers have been infrequent in recent years. "But with good friends that doesn't seem to matter," Don said.

Bob Steadward can claim more than three decades of friendship with Gary, dating from the Edmonton Games for the Physically Disabled. Although in his role as president of the International Paralympic Committee, Bob has travelled the world, often meeting with heads of state, he claims "I would sooner be with [Gary] than any of those people because of what he offers in terms of friendship, intuitiveness, integrity, understanding, tolerance and wisdom."

27 | Gary Today

Two things in life are great teachers: the first is adversity, no matter what form it comes in, and the second is kids. I've been blessed with both.

—GARY McPHERSON [1]

NOTHING ABOUT THE OUTSIDE of Gary and Val McPherson's home suggests that one of its residents is seriously disabled. A basketball hoop stands on the driveway of the ordinary-looking house—there's not a ramp nor a railing in sight. But hidden inside the double garage is a 2000 GMC Savana van fitted with a special hydraulic ramp and an automated platform that can raise a wheelchair from the garage floor to the front hall of the house.

On a recent fall day little white-haired Chester began to sound off as soon as the doorbell rang, playing watchdog, though I doubted if any burglar would be deterred by his high-pitched barking. On entering I was greeted by his wagging tail; we had become friends over the past couple of years. I removed my coat and entered the combined living-dining-computer room, the latter component located on the shortened vertical arm of the T-shaped room.

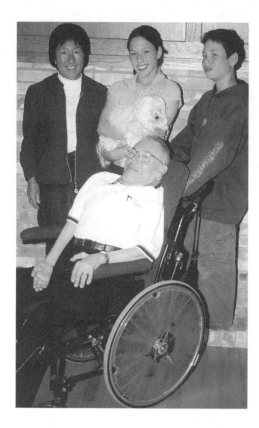

Val, Keiko, Jamie and Gary, the McPherson family in 2003.

Gary sat in his wheelchair, his face five centimetres from the microphone and his eyes fixed on the computer screen. This was his turf, his base of operations, the air traffic control centre of his various and sundry activities. After a couple of quick commands into the microphone, he pushed himself away from the computer desk with his left leg, turned and greeted me with a "Hey, how are y'?"

He looked great, healthy and fit. His twinkling blue eyes and ready smile suggested a wholesome and lively inner state. I found it hard to think of him as disabled. That perception of disability has long since vanished, not just because of familiarity but more because of his great mountain of abilities. His face and neck muscles moved animatedly and expressively, though his right leg did not move at all and his right hand lay motionless on his right thigh, a pale palm facing upwards like a belly-up fish. But he had enough push in his left leg to whip his wheelchair around and just enough movement in his left hand to click the mouse of his computer. He could lean forward a few degrees in his wheelchair and, every now and then, wiggle his torso to relieve pressure areas on his back and rear.

In due course Val came along, put her arm around Gary's shoulder and gave him a drink of water from a straw. He's committed himself to drinking eight glasses of water a day. Joanne, his present attendant who is now on reduced hours, stooped down and emptied his pee-bag. Twelve-year-old Keiko breezed in, waved "hi" and headed for the kitchen; soon afterwards Jamie arrived home from school with a pal. He received a pretty firm "no" in reply to his request to play games on the computer, then headed off to other activities. The phone rang several times during my visit, usually for Gary; he has three ways of answering calls, including a sideways knock with his knee that has the effect of lifting the receiver. Life seemed full, and it felt like a home where people cared. I soon found myself sipping tea and munching one of Val's tasty date squares.

I had to come to ask Gary about his current activities. I knew that he was much in demand as a speaker, based on his uniqueness as a person who had overcome the effects of disability and established a career, raised a family and served his community. His recent speaking engagements included one on handling personal change, given at a Family and Community Support Services conference in Jasper, and "an inspirational talk to the Lupus Society, Edmonton chapter, on the importance of volunteers in our society."

"I understand you have given talks on employing disabled people," I said.

"Last year I spoke on that subject for the Alberta Vocational Counsellors before an audience of six hundred able-bodied people at Grant MacEwan College. It's an important subject because the labour pools in this province are not keeping up with the demand for trained people. One of the potential sources to meet the need is disabled people. They may be more desirable to hire than those who have been on welfare. Bob Chelmick and I worked as a team for this presentation. It was a highly interactive session with many people asking questions. There's still a fair bit of discomfort with disabled employees, and the employees themselves are often a bit naive in making themselves employable. But I honestly believe that progress is being made."

Another recent presentation combined his favourite subject, health, with technology. "Technology has changed the lives of almost everyone, and usually for the better. I am certainly grateful for it. Without respirators I would not be alive and without electronic communications, including my voice-activated computer, my little sphere of activities would shrink to the confines of this room. Yet it is my observation that many working in high technology fields are driven, consumed with the passion to succeed whatever the cost. Their physical, spiritual and emotional health is sacrificed at the altar of 'success.' By the time they are ready to curtail their high-powered careers, many have lost their health, their peace of mind and their family. Sometimes it takes a stroke or a severe heart attack to teach them the lesson they need."

"What about that short course you taught in the MBA program at the university?"

"During that two-day course, George de Rappard and I spoke on 'Effective Meetings for Effective Decision Making' and 'Effective Speaking for Effective Decisions.' It was very well received, so well in fact that we have been asked to repeat it twice next year."

When Keiko returned, dressed in soccer attire, I was reminded of the game her team had played the previous year, which I watched from the sidelines with Val and Gary, alternately cheering or moaning. Gary had become a real supporter of this sport, which he once derided. "I am now the director of soccer for Riverbend [community] with a program involving 1,460 kids from the age of six to eighteen. It all started when a member of the executive phoned and asked if I would come on board as secretary. I have always declined a writing job because I can't write and take minutes, but with the computer voice technology, I no longer had an excuse.

"Ten months later the director resigned, and I was asked to fill his shoes. I just couldn't say no—so many kids, including our own, benefit from soccer. Besides, I think it's fair to say that I have a few organizational skills that could be used here. This past year I was on a steep learning curve, you can be sure. I've always tried to promote volunteerism; my volunteer time right now is primarily in the area of community league soccer."

I knew that Gary had authored or co-authored many papers and articles while he was with the Premier's Council on the Status of Persons with Disabilities, including the regular column in *Status Report*. "Any current writing projects?" I asked.

"Right now I'm co-authoring a chapter for a forthcoming book entitled the *Canadian Handbook on Physical Activity*. It takes in wheelchair sport, sport and disability, fitness, lifestyle and the adaptations that are required to allow people to partake in physical activity at a meaningful level."

Currently Gary is executive-director of the Canadian Centre for Social Entrepreneurship (CCSE) at the University of Alberta. "I'm also an adjunct professor in the Faculty of Physical Education, where I do some guest lecturing on such topics as social, physical and spiritual well-being. But my main commitment is to the CCSE, which was officially launched on November 2, 1999, as a brand-new venture."

"Can you explain in simple terms the function of the CCSE and what you hope to achieve?" I asked.

"The word *entrepreneur* usually applies to business and means seeking opportunity with a bit of risk-taking. Social entrepreneurship means the using of good business principles by people in business, but for the benefit of society. You may be surprised that our new centre is located in the Faculty of Business—business, culturally, is foreign to social concerns.

"We are trying to get more corporations to be socially conscious and responsible. It's altruistic, and we're not ashamed to admit it. I've noticed that some of the MBA students have come back from overseas international experience as changed people. They are asking: 'How can I take what I'm learning in business and apply it for the betterment of mankind?'

"The idea of 'social entrepreneurship' has really taken off in the United States and part of Britain, but it's fairly new in Canada. Last month in Toronto we had an excellent meeting with business leaders, including the CEOs of Toronto Hydro and Syncrude. Eric Newell, CEO of Syncrude and also chairman of the board of governors of the university, is enthused about the idea."

As well, Gary said the CCSE had "received expressions of support and interest from the minister of Alberta Economic Development and his department. Our hope is that the government will see the economic development potential in the whole idea—that social entrepreneurship is about creating economic opportunity as well as contributing towards the betterment of our communities.

"I don't like to look too far down the road—an attitude that's probably the residue from my precarious teenage years. Social entrepreneurship is a relatively new concept that makes very good sense economically and socially, but it won't take off until people have been educated and shown its great value. We are fortunate to have the solid support of the dean of the business faculty and of several business leaders."

At that moment Val arrived to guide me down to the basement room to inspect Gary's lonely collection of honours and awards. When we returned, my mind had drifted back in time. I had never before seen so many certificates, trophies and laurels in one household. I thought about all the energy and versatility and drive that earned this incredible collection of tributes and accolades.

Where did it all come from? Gary's grade two teacher, having followed his career over the years, commented that he had "walked through life to the full." The achievements he chalked up during a sparkling career were nothing less than astounding.

I would never have the temerity to analyze the person of Gary McPherson; his depth and complexity defy analysis—far better to simply let the record speak for itself. Gary is quick to give credit for his growth and intellectual development to his dear friend Clayton, to the Jaycees, to interaction with all kinds of people including hospital staff and wheelchair athletes, and to his involvement with committees, boards and administrative bodies of all kinds. Perhaps these claims contain a lot of truth, but transcending it all is an irrepressible human spirit. Adrienne Riley, pitcher for the slow-pitch ball team that Gary coached, believes he has "a flame burning inside him."

Before leaving, I asked Gary about certain objects in the modest living room. The inukshuk, a configuration of piled stones used by the Inuit as a landmark in hunting caribou, was a gift from Bob and Laura Steadward when Gary received his honorary degree in 1995. "Something like that warms my heart," he said, "because it is an expression of love and caring. So does that painting over there on the wall. It was painted by mouth by my old buddy Henri Baril. And those copper earrings I gave to Betty Fraser for Christmas when I was eleven or so. A few years ago, Betty came over to our house with the earrings; she wanted to give them to Keiko."

A veritable litany of things fill Gary's heart with gratitude, revived each morning when he wakes up. He feels blessed with life itself, with all the people who have enriched his life, for the army of volunteers who have helped him along the way. He is so grateful for his family, for all the activities he has taken part in, for the privilege of living in a great country. He is thankful for work to do and for his unique life story, which can be used to help others, especially those with disabilities.

Asked about his philosophy for day-to-day living, Gary said, "I rarely think about being disabled. I try to focus on today, the projects that I'm working on, the things I can do for my family. I really want to be the best dad and husband I can possibly be, to give them care and affection and to get away from my own self-interest. I try to act out my convictions, but without bulldozing or ignoring others' advice and/or criticism. Because health—emotional, physical and spiritual—is so important, I feel compelled to tell my story and share my views on fitness in order to help other people."

"You have quoted the famous words of Roger Bannister, the great British runner who was the first to break the four-minute mile in 1954: 'The man who can drive himself further once the effort gets painful is the man who will win.' Do those words still inspire you?"

"I think that many athletes, including runners, have to endure pain. In fact, runners can't escape it. For me, persistence has a higher claim. Calvin Coolidge had it about right when he said 'Persistence and determination alone are the omnipotent'. "

As I was leaving, I asked Gary the question that Ron Fortin had posed when they were on a plane together, heading to a wheelchair basketball tournament: "If someone could work the magic and make you an able-bodied person again, would you go for it?"

"I'm not sure," he replied. "I might not choose to do so, because it would mean that all the efforts I have made to reach the place I am in today would be all washed away. It would just be too high a price to pay."

With an envious record behind him, Gary could easily rest on his laurels, content with a job well done. But instead, while he enjoys the present, he looks to the future. A few years ago, he confided to the *Edmonton Journal*'s Cam Tait, "I haven't done my best work yet."

Epilogue

Gifts Given and Lives Touched

Life is no brief candle to me. It is a sort of splendid torch which I have got hold of for the moment, and I want to make it burn as brightly as possible before handing it on to future generations.

——GEORGE BERNARD SHAW

FROM THE BEGINNING Gary was a "mover and a shaker." In elementary school he organized games and sports, even for the older kids. Newly emerged from the iron lung, he learned how to sass the nurses in a raspy voice by manoeuvring a finger to cover his tracheotomy opening. Later, he and Clayton were "mobilizing the forces," organizing a sort of conspiracy to confront hospital administration. They wielded remarkable power, these teenaged boys with wasted, useless arms and legs, and breathing systems that barely sustained life.

Yet, far from being self-serving, there was something admirable about them all, including the youngest: Gary McPherson. Lorraine Habekost claimed that her daughter, Tana, decided to train in respiratory therapy "because of Gary." Lee Sanderson called him "a master of manipulation," but when the time came for her to choose a career, she chose nursing; Gary and his buddies were a major influence in her decision. Gary's first major endeavour, which touched the lives of thirty-one others on the polio ward, was the 1976 "Project Hawaii." The logistics posed a phenomenal challenge, with the need for careful planning down to the most minute details. But lives were changed, and the health and morale of the ward-bound patients took an upward turn in Hawaii. For Gary, the greatest reward was in seeing the pleasure the jaunt gave to others.

His work on behalf of people with disabilities began with the example he presented as a disabled person himself. His own behaviour and friendly talk put people at ease. In fact, many testified that within five minutes of meeting Gary, they somehow found themselves overlooking his physical state. Multiplied by the thousands over the years, such one-on-one incidents effectively changed the way able-bodied people regard those using wheelchairs. Gary thinks he did some of his best advocacy work during the course of the Governor General's Study Conference, when he lived with a small group of able-bodied people for ten days. They lugged his wheelchair up and down stairs and into school buses and learned all about his respirator. Towards the end, they refused to go into a building "if we can't take Gary in with us." Randy Dickinson reported how his wife's father "felt very apprehensive" when Gary arrived at the Dickinson home in Fredericton to attend meetings. Within a few days of living under the same roof, they became friends. When Randy's father-in-law learned that he and Gary would be returning to Alberta on the same flight, he said that the thought of travelling with such an experienced airlines traveller made him "feel secure."

Gary stands in the same league as Rick Hansen—both are giants battling for the cause of the disabled. His involvement as co-chairman of the Alberta segment of the great Man in Motion tour in 1986 led to the Alberta government's commitment to setting up the Premier's Council on the Status of Persons with Disabilities. For ten years Gary served as chairman, wrestling with the needs of the blind, the developmentally challenged, persons with cerebral palsy and the physically disabled generally. As a seriously disabled person, he commanded the respect and confidence from the disabled community that an able-bodied person would be denied. He and his colleagues worked tirelessly on such things as employment practices, support for the disabled and access to buildings.

He authored or co-authored a series of discussion papers, including the 1997 classic "From the Welfare State to the State of Well-Being: Towards a Social Vision for Alberta." Today he remains much in demand as a speaker, and he continues to write on disability and related issues. He and Professor Dick Sobsey together wrote an article for the *Archives of Physical and Rehabilitation Medicine*, rebutting Peter Singer's offensive statement that "killing a cat is a more serious moral ill than killing a child with a disability."

During the course of his work for the disabled community, Gary has ruffled feathers and bruised feelings, but, as Bob Steadward pointed out, "outstanding leaders are not universally loved and admired."

Striving towards his goal of being a lifelong learner, Gary has excelled, as many who have followed his career will testify. His record as a teacher, starting with the Jaycees back in 1968, has been one of solid performance. He learned the skills of effective speaking, leadership training, parliamentary procedure and budgeting, then proceeded to pass them on, beginning with talks to nurses at the Royal Alexandra Hospital. After mastering frog-breathing in 1962 after many failed attempts, he went on to teach and encourage others, his efforts culminating in the production of a video of professional calibre, in collaboration with the Aberhart Hospital's respiratory therapy department, which was presented at an international polio conference in St. Louis, Missouri, in 1983. Collaborating with his former Jaycees colleague George de Rappard, he has taught MBA students in the Faculty of Business on such subjects as effective decision making.

His eclectic contributions to various sporting activities have been nothing short of phenomenal. He took a mixed team of slow-pitch ball players and coached them to heights they never dreamed of. Years later, former pitchers, batters and fielders still sing the praises of those halcyon days when they played good competitive ball, and had great fun doing it. "He brought out the best in me," said Adrienne Riley. "It was good for us when we were in our twenties to have come under his influence. He wasn't afraid of anything." For the children of Gary and Carlene Ogletree, he was a wonderful role model. Carlene, who had played ball since age eight, said, "Gary has risen above things that would imprison most people. He himself succeeds and then carries those around him up to another level."

His contribution to sports for the disabled, especially wheelchair basketball, rank among his greatest achievements. Starting in 1972 as president of the Paralympic Sports Association, he went on to serve the Canadian Wheelchair Sports Association for nineteen years in various capacities. For his long record of service, he has received several honours and tributes. Ann Mecklenberg, who worked with Gary on the Commission of Inclusion of Athletes with a Disability, said, "He has had a huge impact on the world of sport for disabled people." Probably one of his greatest feats was his work as general manager in building the Alberta Northern Lights Wheelchair Basketball Society from an obscure bunch of casual recreational players to one of the top teams in North America.

On a par with his sterling record with the Northern Lights was his influence on the lives of the disabled athletes themselves. Ron Minor wasn't exaggerating when he said, "I was a pretty wild fellow and had a monstrous ego." Before he got involved with the team, he had run afoul of the law more than once. Brought up from Lethbridge to play basket-ball, he met a new friend who was not only willing to promote his abilities but also to help him straighten out his rudderless life. Ron's life under-went a radical change of direction. He developed into a leader on the court, a "twenty-point player" who could be counted upon when the pressure was on. He went on to become an outstanding international athlete in track as well. Now happily married with two children, Ron looks back on those days when a pale, skinny guy in a wheelchair changed the life of a muscular athlete. "I had never seen such dedication and loyalty," he said. "There are no words big enough to describe him."

While recovering from a gunshot wound to his back, Randy Wyness left the rehab ward one day feeling dejected and directed his wheelchair down to the polio ward, where he met Gary. "Little was I to know that everything worthwhile I was to do or become in the next twenty-five years I would owe to Gary McPherson." Like Ron Minor, he was drifting aimlessly—until Gary called and invited him to try out for the Northern Lights. Randy made the team, and wheelchair basketball became his life for the next nineteen years. He even made Canada's Olympic team in 1988 and went to Seoul, Korea—although the exciting game the Northern Lights played in Eugene, Oregon, probably remains the highlight of his career. Married with a family and working in Wetaskiwin at a regular job, Randy considers his friendship with Gary the best thing that ever happened to him. "He's made me the person that I am today. When I die, I will rest happily in peace if they put on my tombstone: 'He was a lot like Gary McPherson'."

There is, understandably, a sort of kinship between people who use wheelchairs, whether or not they are athletes. Percy Wickman, a former MLA who has championed the rights of the disabled by advocating for their cause, is not quite as convinced as Gary is of the value of wheel-chair sport. The two have channelled their energies in different directions, but Percy does not hesitate to say of Gary: "I consider him a Canadian hero." Walter Lawrence, paralyzed from the neck down after a diving acci-dent, works as a peer counsellor and mentor at the G.F. Strong Rehab Centre in Vancouver, a place for the rehabilitation of brain- and spinal-injured persons. Walter maintains that "my strength is made perfect in weakness," a claim made nearly two thousand years ago by the apostle Paul. About his friend Gary, he said, "He'll go the extra mile for you."

Rick Hansen's friendship goes back to 1976 when the Canadian Games for the Physically Disabled were held in Cambridge, Ontario. For twenty-eight days in 1986 they were together, off and on, for the Alberta portion of the famous Man in Motion world tour. He calls Gary "the most able guy I've ever met." Rick played with the Vancouver Cable Cars wheel-chair basketball team, who were often staunch opponents of the Alberta Northern Lights. But when he got the news of the great success of the Northern Lights in Eugene, Oregon, he rejoiced too. "We were proud of them, even if we were rivals," he said. He favoured the writing of a book about Gary McPherson because "telling a story about a great person will help people weave some of the content into their lives." Vance Milligan, the paraplegic lawyer who served as Gary's co-chair for the Alberta part of Rick Hansen's Man in Motion tour, which raised more than five million dollars in Alberta alone, said, "I'd like Gary in the trenches with me."

Gary has touched the lives of innumerable people and the rewards have been great, but to him, they don't quite match the happiness and love and integrity of his family. For a man who never envisaged being married, to say nothing of having children, he considers himself incredibly blessed. If life is stable and purposeful for him, it is in large part because of the love and loyalty of Val, Keiko and Jamie. They are likely to be the most valuable part of his legacy. And they are a family of which any father would be proud. If brightness, spontaneity and creativity are portents of things to come, one can see a bright future for Keiko and Jamie.

Gary has been out of the family circle since the age of nine, when he entered hospital with polio in 1955, but his mother, Dorothy, still refers to him as the "rock" of the family. She knew he was probably closer to the polio buddies with whom he shared nearly every hour of his life, but she wanted to keep the family ties strong. She did more than that: she worked closely with Gary for many years through the Canadian Wheelchair Sports Association.

In sisterly style, Kim offered that Gary could be "the bossiest person and a real pain in the butt." But a minute later, she added, "But he's really a great guy and a kind person." Brother Rod said, "He's been a very important mentor in my life. If I ever feel the least bit sorry for myself, I think of him."

Gary's horizons go beyond the world of the disabled and his own family circle to the community in which he lives. His commitment to soccer in Edmonton's Riverbend community and the fifteen hundred or so kids in the program will, in all likelihood, have a lasting influence. His book *With Every Breath I Take* has already reached into the lives of great numbers of people with its sound advice on health—physical, spiritual and emotional. Considering that the author was confined to an institution for thirty-four years and has emerged with a pretty comprehensive understanding of health and wellness, his words should be taken seriously. He has lived in a frail, wasted body for almost fifty years, yet he remains in good health.

His task at the University of Alberta in developing and promoting the Canadian Centre for Social Entrepreneurship is an awesome one, the sort of a challenge that brings out the best in Gary. It's a relatively new venture—to get the business world (and others) to give serious consideration to creating economic opportunity as well as contributing to the betterment of our communities.

Randy Dickinson, chairman of the New Brunswick Premier's Council on the Status of Disabled Persons, said Gary's "level of participation in his community is far beyond that of most able-bodied people. His role in national and international groups, his travel to everywhere in Canada and several foreign countries, his role as a keynote speaker and participant in many national and regional conferences on disability issues and human rights issues and sports concerns—who could ever measure all these?" Russell Carr, an associate of Gary's on the Alberta Premier's Council, believes his greatest contribution has been his effort to clarify and educate others about real health and what it means.

How would Gary like to be remembered? His answer is twofold. First, by his children, as a good father who loved them. And second, as someone who made a contribution.

As this book was going to press, a news release announced that Gary McPherson had been awarded the Order of Canada and was invited to Ottawa in the fall of 2003 to receive the award from Governor General Adrienne Clarkson. Her words capture the essence of an amazing man.

The citation reads as follows:

His story is one of incredible determination. For nearly 35 years, Gary McPherson lived in a long-term care facility after childhood polio left him quadriplegic. Now living independently, he has become a leading social activist, wheelchair athlete and sports administrator, inspiring others with his record of social service. A key player within the Alberta Paraplegic Foundation and the Rick Hansen Centre, among others, he has worked with every level of government to influence public policy and introduce legislation that reflects our commitment to building an inclusive society.

Notes

2 Schoolboy in the Yukon

1 Russell Taylor, *Polio '53: A Memorial for Russell Frederick Taylor* (Edmonton: University of Alberta Press, 1990), 13.

2 Ibid., 46.

3 "Conquering the Crippler," a CBC-TV program which aired Dec. 6, 1993, transcript, 5.

8 The Frog-Breather

1 "Frog Breathing with Gary McPherson," a nine-minute video produced by the Respiratory Therapy Department, Aberhart Centre, University of Alberta Hospital, Edmonton, 1983.

9 Outings Far from the Polio Ward

1 Bob Johnson, "Have Old Yeller, Will Travel," *The Caliper* (Canadian Paraplegic Association: Summer 1965), 5.

10 The Allure of Sports

1 *St. Paul Journal*, June 2, 1982, 1.

13 On the Road and in the Air

1 Harold Lucas Fryer, "Gary McPherson: Travelling Man," *The Caliper* (Fall 1967), 6.

2 "Handicapped Canadians Leave Cold for Dream Trip," *Honolulu Star-Bulletin* (March 4, 1976), C20; "Hawaii Is only a Wheel Away," *Honolulu Advertiser* (March 4, 1976), A1.

3 House of Representatives of the State of Hawaii, House Resolution no. 416, March 16, 1976.

4 President's Dinner, annual meeting of the Alberta Medical Association, September 24, 1976.

15 The Hospital

1 Darryl Rock, *Making a Difference: Profiles in Abilities* (Toronto: Canadian Abilities Foundation, 2001), 71.

16 Wheelchair Basketball and the Great Alberta Northern Lights

1 As quoted in Robert Steadward and Cynthia Peterson, *Paralympics: Where Heroes Come* (Edmonton: One Shot Holdings Publishing Division, 1997), 15.

17 Rick Hansen and the Man in Motion Tour

1 Rick Hansen and Jim Taylor, *Rick Hansen: Man in Motion* (Vancouver: Douglas and McIntyre, 1987), 13.

2 Shelley Gillen, "Rick Hansen Comes Home," *Chatelaine* (June 1987), 81.

20 Premier's Council

1 Alberta Premier's Council on the Status of Persons with Disabilities, *Status Report* (August 1998), 3.

21 A Great Family

1 *Edmonton Journal* (September 29, 1999), G2.

23 Gary McPherson, Author

1 As quoted in Joan L. Hedley, "We Call Ourselves Survivors," *Polio Network News* 10, no. 1 (Winter 1994), 1.

2 Gary McPherson, "A Monkey Shakes the Tree: A New Paradigm for Rehabilitation," paper presented at National Rehabilitation Conference, Halifax, October 1995.

3 Gary McPherson, *With Every Breath I Take: One Person's Extraordinary Journey to a Healthy Life and How You Can Share in It* (Edmonton: Double M Brokerage, 2000), 25.

4 McPherson, *With Every Breath I Take*, 55.

5 Ibid., 126.

6 Ibid., 73.

7 Ibid., 93.

8 Ibid., 87.

24 Stronger by Weakness

1 David Hingsburger on the "Life, Death and Disability" segment of CBC-Radio's "Ideas" program (May 23, 2001). Used with permission.

2 Statements made by Anita Dadson, Gregor Wolbring, Angus McLaren, David Hingsburger, Dick Sobsey and Lucy Gwin are excerpts from the transcript of the CBC-Radio "Life, Death and Disability" program.

3 Alberta Human Rights and Citizenship Commission, *Status Report* (November 1999), 1.

4 Premier's Council on the Status of Persons with Disabilities, *Status Report* (February, 1998), 3.

25 Disabled Heroes

1 As quoted in Charlene Rooke, "After Atlanta: The International Paralympic Committee President Keeps on Building," *New Trail* (University of Alberta alumni magazine; Winter 1996–97), 38.

2 Rick Pilger, "Igniting a Passion for Learning," *New Trail* (Winter 1994–95), 7. The author learned of the sad death of Jim Vargo after completing the writing of this book.

3 Alberta Premier's Council on the Status of Persons with Disabilities, *Status Report* (August 2001), 1.

26 Awards and Friendships

1 The author was recently saddened to learn of Marshall Smith's death.

27 Gary Today

1 As quoted in Steadward et al., *Paralympics: Where Heroes Come*, 215.